Building the Successful
Veterinary Practice

Building the Successful Veterinary Practice

VOLUME 1

Leadership Tools

Thomas E. Catanzaro

DVM, MHA, Diplomate,
American College of Healthcare Executives

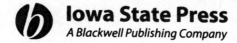

Iowa State Press
A Blackwell Publishing Company

Thomas E. Catanzaro, DVM, MHA, Diplomate, American College of Healthcare Executives, received his DVM from Colorado State University and his master's in healthcare administration from Baylor University. He was the first veterinarian to receive Board certification with the American College of Healthcare Executives. In the last decade Catanzaro, the author of numerous articles, has visited, assisted, or consulted with over 1,200 veterinary practices in the United States, Canada, and Japan.

© 1997 Thomas E. Catanzaro
All rights reserved

No part of this book may be reproduced in any form or by any electronic or mechanical means, including information storage and retrieval systems, without permission in writing from the copyright holder, except for brief passages quoted in review.

⊚ Printed on acid-free paper in the United States of America

First edition, 1997

Library of Congress Cataloging-in-Publication Data

Catanzaro, Thomas E.
 Building the successful veterinary practice: leadership tools / Thomas E. Catanzaro.—1st ed.
     p.   cm.
 Includes bibliographical references (p.   ) and index.
 ISBN 0-8138-2819-8
 1. Leadership. 2. Veterinary medicine—Practice. I. Title.
SF760.L43C37 1997
636.089′068′4—dc21   97-374

Last digit is the print number: 9 8 7 6 5 4 3 2

CONTENTS

EACH OF US is the sum of what we have experienced, whom we have met, and the environment that has guided our destiny. I have five decades of people, places, and communities to recognize and can't include them all. Therefore, I would like to dedicate this book to the veterinary profession.

In the evolution of veterinary practice management, gone are the days of the quick-fix and the gimmick of the moment. We are in an era that requires an integrated set of programs delivered by a dedicated team. Every team needs leadership, and it is the uncommon leader who emerges as the success story in our profession today. The uncommon leader centers on staff harmony, team pride in the practice, and the enhancement of client access. Gone are the days when only strong control by the doctor or the hiring of a process-based manager can develop a market niche.

My wife of 30 years gave me not only two great kids, but also the ability to experience many different practice settings. We moved 17 times in the first 21 years of marriage. (People who know us call her Saint Ann for her tolerance, understanding, and nurturing of our family.) The consulting team we built during the four years I was hospital services director at the American Animal Hospital Association (AAHA) was one such team of uncommon leaders. The associate team of my veterinary practice consultancy is another such team. I am a lucky person. I have found those who care about the profession before themselves, colleagues who place ethics before profits and are willing to sacrifice for others. These are the traits of the uncommon leaders of our profession.

This book is designed to expose the values and skills of a leader in the veterinary profession. Once these values are exposed and classified, veterinary leaders can start to nurture them within themselves and then within their team. The book is designed after numerous leadership courses that I have conducted over the past 12 years in the United States as well as in other nations. The values, techniques, and skills shared in this reference have also proved to be successful in over 1,200 veterinary facilities we've visited during the past seven years. The secret is in the individual, not in this book. When we expose a skill or a concept, readers must find the values and strength within themselves to adapt and change. The ones who read, understand, and embrace the concepts contained herein will become the uncommon veterinary medical leaders of tomorrow, and they are the ones whom this profession will acknowledge as successful.

ACKNOWLEDGMENTS

IMPORTANT CONTRIBUTIONS to this book have been made by many practices and managers I have known and visited as hospital services director of the American Animal Hospital Association and as president of our own full-time, veterinary-exclusive, practice consulting firm. The comprehensive and personal feedback many have offered to hundreds of articles I've written, to common literature in this profession, and to many seminars we have conducted has been very helpful in developing this first volume in a series of leadership texts.

From leadership experience in Vietnam to the Army-Air Force consolidation opportunity to design and put on the ground over 100 veterinary clinic facilities in less than two years, my formative years were diversified. Baylor University's master's in healthcare administration (1983–85) was an academic catalyst, and Dick Harder was a significant mentor during those years. The consulting team we built at AAHA was the first sounding board for these philosophies, and those members need to be acknowledged here: Rosemarie Warren; Terry Hall, DVM; Phil Seibert, CVT; Sandra Hamper, RN, MHA; Jim Shirey, DVM; and John Schiebelhut. They shared a wealth of experience and ideas, many becoming the prime source of our consulting philosophy progress. My companion through all of this was a caring and nurturing person, known as Ann M. Muraski when she was a high-school sweetheart, who became my wife over 30 years ago. She cared for our two children, Michael and Deborah, and ensured they were raised with a respect for life and rights of others—two-legged or four—while I was building administration programs and visiting veterinary hospitals in Japan, Central America, Canada, Europe, and across the United States of America.

The manuscript was assembled from many of my articles and personal literary efforts, and Elizabeth K. Schultz has been tenacious in proofing and rendering readable my attempts at combining many leadership thoughts into a single document. We used the final draft for our *Seminars at Sea '95*, and Elizabeth Schultz also integrated feedback evaluations from participants to improve the flow and readability. In 1996 Gretchen Van Houten and Jane Zaring came onto the scene; they are leaders of the team from Iowa State University Press who evolved all our efforts into this book. No man is an island, and this first of three leadership texts proves that observation. Thanks to one and all.

Building the Successful Veterinary Practice

Nurturing Your Leadership Competencies

Nurture—the act or process of promoting the development of; training.

It is a puzzle faced by every practice leader today: How do you effectively lead a practice team during a time when everything from structure, to community, to strategies, to values is dramatically changing? When do you empower the employees? When do you coach them? When do you direct them? When must you demand? How do you know which style of leadership is needed?

Such leadership strategies have shifted along with everything else, bringing with them confusing and conflicting changes in terminology and techniques. Bombarded with exhortations from the Total Quality Management (TQM) movement of industry, to the Continuous Quality Improvement (CQI) movement of healthcare, to the Total Quality Service/Total Management Service (TQS/TMS) copycat ideas of lateral organizations, compounded by a wide variety of self-appointed management experts, it is no wonder that veterinary practice leaders don't know whether to reengineer their personalities, reinvent the practice organization, or simply become virtuous human beings and try to please everyone in every situation.

Total quality management awareness and training programs have proved successful when the leadership releases accountability for outcomes to the employees. In healthcare this action violates the State Practice Act, so continuous quality improvement has evolved as the alternative. The teams in either case try to improve the organizational processes, which are usually messy interdepartmental problems.

Skill Is Not Enough

Inadequate performance of any practice is rarely due to a lack of knowledge or technical skill. Think about deficient managers you have watched in your own practice. More often than not, their failure or inferior performance in a specific position can be traced to attitudes, motives, style, or personal characteristics they rely on to carry out the responsibilities of their jobs. In some cases the owner has delegated the process without the authority, responsibility, or accountability to make it better; or, worse yet, delegated the job without having provided the training. Understanding the concept of "training to trust" before delegating will be one of our goals for the rest of this lesson.

The Competencies Iceberg

Although technical skills and knowledge are indeed important factors in job success and are the visible portion of the manager's capabilities, they represent only the tip of the iceberg. The rest of the iceberg factors are less obvious. They lie under the surface, but they are the competencies required for superior results within any team.

Competencies can include any trait, behavior, skill, or other personal attribute that permits or nurtures outstanding performance. Although some competencies are relatively easy to train and develop, others are deeply embedded traits of an individual that cannot be changed from the outside, regardless of the good intentions of the trainer. They are personal inner values, learned at an early age or by experience, and can be tuned only by individuals themselves. The best of leaders and trainers can nurture the changes, but they can directly affect only the environment. Mothers know it, scoutmasters practice it—and it is *Behavior rewarded is behavior repeated.* The leader nurtures development (self and others) by rewarding the positive. In the quest to modify these inner values of others, the savvy leader sets up discoveries, or capitalizes on an actual event, to gain cognitive awareness by a team member of a need to modify attitudes, behavior, traits, motives, social roles, or other leadership competencies.

The skills and knowledge of the Competencies Iceberg are what appear on the resume, and what most veterinarians screen for during candidate

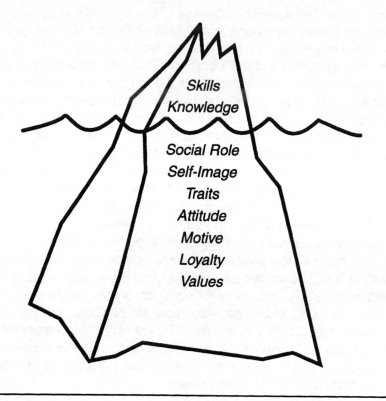

Skills

Knowledge

Social Role

Self-Image

Traits

Attitude

Motive

Loyalty

Values

Fig. I.1. Graphic representation of the Competencies Iceberg

interviews. But if the person being added to the team is not screened for the underlying competencies, the search will be conducted again in a few months because the person didn't fit the team or because, uncomfortable with the environment, the person left. This same principle applies to leadership and managers already in the practice. The competencies that lie below the surface will be the real determining factors for superior performance, team harmony, and practice success.

How a Leader Nurtures

Nurturing the competencies in self and others is leadership in action and an operational key to less stress and more harmony!

Although it is difficult to predict which leadership competencies will be important in the future of any specific veterinary practice, we can look to the history of successful healthcare organizations and seek models of excellence. In fact, The American College of Healthcare Executives (ACHE) has shown that leadership—not staff—makes CQI or TQM programs succeed or fail. Uncommon leaders are required to make CQI a successful process. The systematic identification of different competencies makes a competency model more than a simple list of desired attributes and qualities. But a disclaimer is required, even with this approach. In the landmark text of a decade ago, *In Search of Excellence,* 10 industries were held up as excellent models, but as we entered the 1990s, half of those had fallen on hard times. They had not changed with the society and community they supported. Leadership and excellence are dynamic. Change is the rule, not the exception, and what worked yesterday may likely not work tomorrow. The true leader is rare, but uncommon leadership is what the future requires for continued success in veterinary medicine.

The competencies that lead to superior performance in one practice may or may not lead to superior performance in another. Every veterinary organization has its own culture, distinct challenges, and unique environment. Although labels and general descriptions may be the same—*team, leadership, harmony, innovation*—the specific behavior indicators will be very different from practice to practice. This is why it is so important to observe and study what people are actually doing to achieve the results considered superior in our profession. Given these parameters, it is possible to develop a core set of competencies.

Core Set of Competencies

These competencies have been selected and modified to reflect the unique challenges inherent in veterinary practice leadership.

Vision
- The Vivid Dream—paints the dream so vividly with words that all around him/her have no doubt where the goal will be.
- Strategic Orientation—develops and maintains a broad-based, long-term perspective on the mission and the business of veterinary medicine.
- Conceptual—quickly grasps the connection between diverse ideas, concepts, issues, and events, never blaming others, but rather looking for the internal cause-and-effect relationships.
- Analytical—breaks down complex problems, tasks, and projects into manageable, logically related components that team members can understand, share ideas about, and develop alternatives for.

Leadership
- Drive—shows an intense personal desire for excellence, wants to lead

and motivate others to excel and grow.

- Change—embraces new ideas, expects innovation and creativity, wants people to solve problems at their level, champions continuous quality improvement in every practice aspect and job position.
- Harmony—models effective leadership in personal behavior, is predictable and dependable, exhibits confidence in staff's ability as well as in the individual expertise of team members.
- Trust—shows respect, gives responsibility and accountability for outcomes, recognizes risk takers, gives credit and takes the blame.

Practice

- Organizational Understanding—identifies specific dysfunctional operations, changes job to fit the strengths of the individual, sees process as secondary to client-centered outcomes.
- Talent—promotes for performance and productivity, not tenure; focuses on staff development and training on a recurring basis; communicates performance expectations based on developmental growth.
- Ownership—encourages involvement and accountability by including lowest staff level possible in decision making; encourages initiative, self-direction, and unilateral decisions based on what is right for the situation.
- Belonging—fosters a sense of being needed and trusted at all levels, considers competency a daily goal, recognizes and appreciates participation on a daily basis.

Results

- Achievement—continually strives to maximize limited resources to achieve higher-quality results for client and patient.
- Bias for Action—balances need for consensus and involvement with the need for decisiveness and action, believes "luck" is being ready to grab an opportunity as it passes by.
- Accountability—provides clear and specific expectations for outcomes, holds self and staff accountable to agreed-upon goals and objectives, accepts personal accountability for poor levels of training expertise within team.
- Recognition—seeks to commend unique and creative actions, tailors the reward to the individual, makes practice improvement contests fun and ensures at least 60 percent of the staff can be winners.

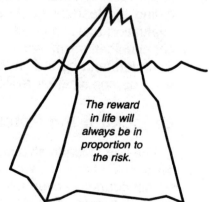

The reward in life will always be in proportion to the risk.

Self-Action
- Self-Confidence—projects strong belief in own ideas and abilities without being arrogant.
- Responsibility—internally accepts accountability for everything that affects the practice; does not blame others inside or outside the practice; is accountable for solutions, not excuses.
- Commitment—aligns personal priorities and behavior with the mission, balances home life and practice, yields personal bias to the good of the practice and/or client.
- Insight—exhibits desire and openness to learn from others and from experience, continually works toward growth and development of self and interteam relationships.

Levels of Leadership

Although these definitions provide a general framework for relevant leadership competencies, they do not include the level of behavioral detail required for accurate measurement and development guidance that differs significantly from practice to practice. Table I.1 reflects the yardstick used to measure the development of the uncommon leader needed in veterinary practice today.

The levels 1 to 12 reflect an increasing proficiency in team leadership. When someone classifies his or her comfort zone as an 8 or a 9, the numbers between that rating and 12 reflect competencies and traits that need to be pursued, nurtured, and practiced. The comfort zone must be stretched with recurring applications of new skills and competencies until they become the new standard.

Some practice leaders do not have an accurate mirror to look into on a regular basis. They need to develop a survey, using the competency models, the levels scale, and, most often, an outside consultant skilled in leadership assessment. The survey is for staff and associates to use in targeting the leadership style(s) most often seen in the practice day. This evaluation tool is a good team builder *if* the boss is willing to listen. Good communications means the ability to listen, to hear what is being said, and to understand no one in the practice really wants to hurt its success, as each person's career relies upon the practice becoming better.

Unlocking the Potentials

The key to leadership growth and development is accurate and focused feedback. I know too well, having been an instructor of over a dozen leadership courses—over half of which were in a high-adventure, outdoor format—that the quality of performance feedback is inversely related to one's

Table I.1. The development of the uncommon leader

12	**LEADS**—has genuine charisma
11	Positions self as leader, ensures everyone buys into mission, oversees group tasks
10	Acts to protect group, gathers right people, resources, and information for the team
9	Uses complex strategies to promote teamwork and cooperation in hiring and discipline decisions, team assignments—cross-training required
8	Uses power and authority in fair and equitable manner
7	Publicly gives credit to others; encourages and empowers others; promotes friendly climate, good morale, and cooperation
6	**FACILITATES**—Values others' input and expertise, ensures everyone contributes, encourages initiative
5	Expresses positive expectations of others, speaks of subordinates in positive manner, respects others and appeals to their reason
4	Keeps people informed and up-to-date; clear, concise expectations.
3	**MANAGES**—Oversees meetings and projects; states agendas and objectives, controls time, and makes assignments; trains to task
2	Cooperates, participates willingly
1	**PARTICIPATES**—Becomes involved reluctantly, suffers burnout, a footdragger
0	Neutral-passive, does not participate—abdicates
-1	Disruptive, uncooperative, causes conflict and disharmony

organizational level. But those barriers are broken down when an outside facilitator enters the group. The higher you are, the less truth people are willing to share about your behavior and attitude. In fact, for a veterinary practice owner, an association executive director, or even a practice administrator, you are very vulnerable to misleading and inaccurate input regarding personal style, cognitive ability, leadership effectiveness, or organizational savvy.

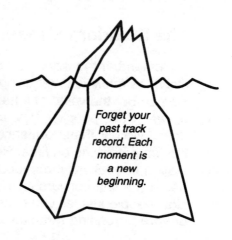

Forget your past track record. Each moment is a new beginning.

The competencies described in this section will provide a head start in developing a plan and process that will ensure meaningful and relevant goals. If the staff is nurtured and rewarded for participating in the new developmental process, feedback quality will improve and the leader will become better. As leadership improves, so does the delegation and sharing of accountability by the team. As the team accepts accountability, responsibility, and ownership for their corner of the practice, the continuous quality improvement and problem prevention will become the standard. Progress will replace status quo, change will replace inertia, and net growth will replace gross growth without net. Times will be easier, the team will be happier, and stress will come into perspective.

Redesigning Leadership

There is one mark of a true leader ... followers!
—Dr. T. E. Cat

There are not many courses in schools that teach kids how to make mistakes, how to weather rough moments, or how to be innovative. Creativity, tenacity, and latitude are required when breaking the rules to make the phoenix rise from the ashes. The traditional "do it this way" attention to process causes stagnation and frustration in a changing environment. The status quo provides comfort, but it also inhibits capturing opportunity. This status quo habit can be referred to as "waiting for the phoenix" mythology. In veterinary practice, success is the ability to adapt to the changing environment, differentiating the practice in the eyes of clients, or developing a unique market niche. That is why we don't see it too often. It requires an uncommon leadership to make change the practice norm.

The Standard Measurement

Remember the day when a person's word was his or her bond? Our society has evolved to requiring a legal written contract that is loophole free. Remember the value of a handshake, when it was a commitment to keep between two people? Now commitment is expected to be listed in a job description, with performance standards, and with extra productivity pay if the job gets done on time. Remember the clerk at the corner store or gas station in your neighborhood who not only knew your name but remembered the last conversation you shared, and then asked how you were? Now people just tell you to keep the line moving. Nostalgia for those days of yore is running rampant lately. Everyone knows something is missing (humanness), but most don't know how to regain it. The veterinary practice leaders who establish these old, yet new, commitments to people and their feelings are the ones that are becoming more successful in today's competitive market.

The uncommon leader accepts the role as having only two functions: (1) to cause things to happen (get the task done), and (2) to create an atmosphere wherein people can come together and achieve professional and personal success (keep the group together). This uncommon leader adapts critical principles of credibility and humanness to the situation at hand, keeps the group moving forward together, and helps the group accomplish the task with a flair and pride with which all can identify.

Some of the most common standards of uncommon leadership are:

Create a Shared Vision

Reality is in the eye of the beholder. It cannot be mandated unless the atmosphere is driven by fear and intimidation. Even then, it doesn't hold the team together. Good people will abandon the leader who is a bully. When we put the receptionist in charge of the appointment log, or the technician in charge of the treatment day sheet, practice effectiveness increases. Less secure doctors fear losing the approval process, but they never improve the system for the operators, so they are not losing anything except efficiency.

Creating a shared vision takes time. It requires the uncommon leader to practice reflective questioning with the staff rather than to use the traditional "I have a great idea" approach. When the process gets rough, when the budget gets tight, when the time line is being extended, the uncommon leader resists snapping back to the authoritarian dictatorship that first created the practice. Shared vision may start with one person making a decision (a staff member emphasizing quality and equality), or the group deciding what the community really needs from a veterinary practice. The key is to start.

Establish Credibility

This is a one-shot process. It is not a short-term, quick fix program of the month. Blow it once and you have years of uphill road repair just to get back to where you started. Most people have been abused by teachers or employers before they join a veterinary healthcare delivery team. They accept the fact that

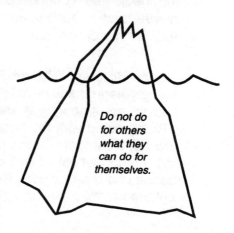

Do not do for others what they can do for themselves.

management promises yet seldom delivers unless the boss can gain personally. Once burned, twice shy. The problem is not the words, not the plan, not the vision: it is the scars. The first error, the unhappy client, the staff friction—the uncommon leader uses these as learning opportunities rather than reactions or reasons for reversion to an authoritarian approach. Credibility is not knee jerking, it is resisting top-down management decisions and showing trust in the team to make things right. Credibility is supporting each person's commitment to excellence, practice harmony, and client-centered service.

Encourage Risk Taking

Creative thinking and visionary planning are critical strengths when you try to break the status quo. The team members will step beyond known ground *only* when they know their leader is their cheerleader. New ideas cause new energies, especially when they come from the staff. Every practice needs to replace "no" with "try it" and replace the limits with encouragement to make changes. The concept of continuous quality improvement says each person must be accountable for changing any part of the process that he or she touches to improve the outcome. Get rid of the blame, plan to make mistakes, and celebrate the effort of trying new ideas.

Be Authentic

Even the most uncommon leader has weaknesses as well as strengths, and the best will personally let his or her team know where the leader needs special help. The first complaint from the traditional practice owner is, "I can't give up the control (I'd be vulnerable)." This is the fright common to the old guard—and the excitement common to the uncommon leader. Change requires letting go; it requires believing in the caring, dedicated, compassionate nature of the staff; but most of all, it requires trust in each team member. Never hide the fact that you need help from a caring team.

Promote Honesty Without Fear

Many veterinarians have killed their practice by promoting and nurturing yea-sayers among their staff. Too many practice staffs equate security with agreeing with the boss. Sharing blame and the fear of retribution are not what fuel practice pride (pride is what clients perceive as quality). An honest opinion is just as important as taking a calculated risk on behalf of a practice goal. Risk taking and honesty are the hot prods that get the practice moving again. Telling the truth, admitting mistakes, and open feedback must be common and celebrated to make coming to work a comfortable process.

Keep Communication Real

The computer does not bill someone—you do. The days of treating people as required interfaces with your computer system are over. The computer age has made consumers smarter. They can recognize this mind-set—including the preprinted label of the preprinted pet-loss sympathy card—for the communication shutdown that it truly is. Automated sympathy does not count. "Business is business" has a place in all healthcare facilities, but not in patient care or client-centered services. Personalities cannot be ignored ... likes, hopes, and fears are real. Take the time to be human, to care, to hear what is meant rather than to react to what is said.

The uncommon leader lets the person (staff or client) finish his or her statements *before* beginning to formulate a reply. Listening to the personal side is often called diplomacy, but it is actually forming a relationship. In multishift practices a *handwritten memo* is far more effective than *establishing a new policy*, especially when rewarding appropriate behavior by saying thanks.

Accommodate Spontaneity

A busy practitioner doesn't usually have time to listen to clients or to staff. When things get slower, the habits have been formed and there still isn't time. The leadership gets out of touch with staff and client needs, and single-brain thinking sets the practice course. Anyone who ever had a study group, a mentor, or an effective task force knows that synergy between two or three brains causes outcomes far better than a single-brain process. There must always be time to listen. Idea exchange must occur when the opportunity arises if creative energy is to be maintained. Remember ARF—Absolute Rigid Flexibility; lots of flex is critical, especially if you want people to know you care enough to listen.

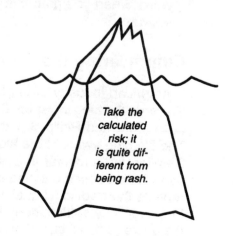

Take the calculated risk; it is quite different from being rash.

Care About the Irritants

The number and seriousness of an individual's gripes are directly and inversely related to the amount of quality improvement energy that the staff member is likely to put into the practice. Personal peeves are a leader's golden fleece. They need to be tracked down, brought into the open, and resolved. When management defines a problem out of existence, it remains and saps the life energy from the team. When staff members know the leader is listening, that knowledge affects their sense of well-being. A happy team begins to emerge. A happy team enhances the services and products they provide; market share improvements occur with spontaneity.

Support Personal and Family Values

There is no such thing as a conflict between home and work; there are only dual standards, as the doctors usually have the right to take off and handle their personal problems, whereas the staff does not. Human decisions are not just to be tolerated. They are to be expected and encouraged. Virtually every veterinary staff member is conscientious to a fault. They don't take advantage, they play fair. When you treat associates' personal lives with respect and caring, they treat the clients and other staff with respect and caring.

Continuous Improvement

Growth requires change, change requires focus on the vision, focus on the vision requires commitment by the individual, individual efforts require the leadership to focus on what the intent was based upon, and the uncommon leader understands that people make decisions because of a caring heart. Each person must feel accountable for change, accountable for making next week better than this week, accountable for improving each client encounter. This can only be done person by person, starting with the uncommon leader. The talk must be seen in the walk! When you grab this tiger by the tail, get ready for an uncommon energy.

Empowering the Person

American industry talks of Total Quality Management: the effects of W. Edwards Deming in Japan, the impact of Joseph M. Juran on American industry, and the Philip S. Crosby books, which make TQM easy to read. The Deming award is the highest quality award in Japan. Most forget that Deming had a mentor at Bell Laboratories, Walter Shewhart, the first person who proposed creating a continuous cycle of improvement that would replace the traditional quality control efforts of America. Deming refined it to a simplicity seldom seen in industry: focus on the average worker and the average product, not on the outliers. Blame the system established by the corporation, not the individual. Drive fear out of the organization and replace it with education and trust.

If a beaver used the traditional quality control approach to building a dam on a river, he would set minimum standards and have a few friends act as managers while other beavers built a few reasonable-looking dams just as they were directed to do. In the places where the initial dams were breached, the material or workmanship would be rejected by a head supervisory beaver. The busy beavers responsible would be admonished. Percentages would guarantee that at least one dam held, and the CEO beaver would quickly sell or lease it for some tasty aspen bark. It is to the environment's benefit that beavers don't work like that. They are into continuous quality improvement. They attack problems at their source and redesign as they go along. They make sure each dam is not only acceptable, but that it provides the desired outcome: a pond to support and protect the lodge. Beavers have standards, an outcome vision that makes them busily work toward excellence, and they stay accountable for that outcome for their entire life.

Getting leaders to shift their focus from blaming individuals to blaming the processes will not work if the staff are excluded from the picture. At human hospitals, where the quality thrust has gone astray, one or more of three factors have been present. First, the leadership has not walked the talk. Quality improvement was delegated to others to implement. Second, the emphasis was on the importance of the new system, which invariably deemphasized the importance of the individual. Third, quality concepts were introduced as a new program, with a beginning, middle, and end. People could wait it out. A continuous quality improvement commitment is forever, and those who believe "And this too shall pass" will die in their procrastination. Once founded in clear values and bioethical principles, the CQI process will not be stopped by any force. Staff who cause change, or just take the risks to attempt change, are celebrated. The staff who fight for the status quo are starved from existence.

The answer to a practice's problems is the people themselves. The leader is responsible for the environment, the tone of the practice atmosphere. If productivity and morale are low, the leader is not taking the right steps. But it is never a single person who controls the practice atmosphere. The leader establishes the mood, and the team creates the processes and systems that get the work done. "Empowerment" is a term often used but not often defined. In most

If it is to be, it's up to me!

practices it can be defined as *caring enough to confront*. This confrontation feedback is an important value at the center of the staff-doctor relationship. It is a trait to be respected and cherished.

■ ■ ■ Review ■ ■ ■

Now that we've given you the philosophy of this course, let us recap the information.

1. KSA—Knowledge, Skills, Attitude—occupy your own space!

2. The uncommon leader has two functions:
   a. Cause things to happen—organize success
   b. Create a successful atmosphere for team participation

3. The most common standards of measurement of uncommon leadership are:
   a. Create a shared vision
   b. Establish credibility
   c. Encourage risk taking
   d. Be authentic
   e. Promote honesty without fear
   f. Keep communication real
   g. Accommodate spontaneity
   h. Care about the irritants
   i. Support personal and family values
   j. Seek continuous improvement
   k. Empower people

4. The core competencies for success are based upon five factors:
   a. Vision—the dream, forward orientation, concepts, and analysis
   b. Leadership—drive, change, harmony, trust
   c. Practice—understanding, using talents, giving ownership, belonging
   d. Results—achievement, action, accountability, recognition
   e. Self-action—self-confidence, responsibility, commitment, insight

5. Standards to measure the uncommon leader include:
   a. Shared vision
   b. Credibility
   c. Risk taking
   d. Authenticity

e. Honesty without fear
f. Effective communication
g. Spontaneity
h. How irritants are treated
i. Personal/family values
j. Continuous improvement

CHAPTER ONE

The Foundation

Attitude of a Leader

The team effort is a lot of people doing what I say ... NOT!

We often hear about the importance of being a good team player, but the term seems to be a cliche, as rarely are the qualities of a good team player defined. As we were raised in America, most of us have played a team sport. It seems to be a requirement in the American school system. Some excelled, but most of us were just good team members. We have all known poor team members: poor sports who had to have it their way, or wanted to be the star and didn't have the talent or training. We also remember the great team members, the ones who made us feel good just to share the game with them. They encouraged us while we learned and let us star when we were ready mentally and physically. Generally, this is the image we think of when we say "team player."

There are always good players, but good players are not always good team members. Remember the ball hog? Remember the pitcher who wouldn't listen to his catcher's signals? The soccer player who would pass laterally only as a panic reaction, or the volleyball player who never would set you up? That volleyball player could have been the best spiker on the net, but it didn't make you want to play another game. A good team player usually sacrifices personal glory for the good of the team.

The analogy to sport activities is only a start, but don't get confused. Seldom does a sport involve life-and-death decisions, rarely does overtime start after eight hours of demanding effort or even the 10- to 12-hour push days, and there is no free substitution when someone is having a bad day. Veterinary practice is not a game, and you are accountable for the outcome of each event, not just for a position. So let's take a look at what the experts in business relations identify as the qualities of a good team player.

Definition of a Team Player

A willingness to sacrifice for the benefit of the team

For a healthcare team to be successful, the personalities must merge into one working unit. Yes, the doctor's license is on the line, but seldom is this an issue. Staff harmony, patient care, and a client-centered focus are the primary issues. When you are part of a healthcare team, the emphasis is not on personal recognition, but on the patient, and that is the way it should be. An exception may occur when you have a specialist group, a surgeon mentality, which brings the clients in because of a name. If you are a good team player, lack of personal recognition or working with a star specialist won't bother you. You will be happy to bask in the glory of the practice and in the recognition the entire team gets in doing a job well.

A willingness to let the team leader lead

This may sound unusual, but many practices hinder the middle managers by restricting their leadership latitude from either the top down or the bottom up. You should be willing to let the team leader guide the group. If you absolutely cannot work for a team leader, say so at the onset and be ready to work elsewhere. Just as you were chosen for your special skills, the team leader was identified for an attitude and skills the leadership thought were appropriate. When the leadership has decided to trust an individual with directing the team or part of the team, your choice is to support that leader 110 percent or resign and move elsewhere.

The ability to contribute your best as a team member

It is not uncommon to hear someone say he or she can do something better (or faster) alone, but this is not the attitude that builds a team. Maybe someone has always been a loner and doesn't work well as part of a team. If this is the case, help that person get out of veterinary healthcare as soon as possible. When someone joins a veterinary healthcare delivery team, even under protest, that person must contribute his or her best efforts. Each team member was hired for an expertise that will help the team, provide better patient care, or keep clients coming back to the practice. Ex-

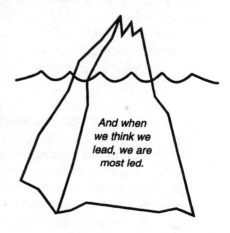

And when we think we lead, we are most led.

pect each team member to do his or her best to make all three things occur. If someone is going to be in conflict with the team leader, ensure that the practice's directing veterinarian has sanctioned the split away from the principles mentioned in number 2.

A spirit of compromise

Teams usually make decisions by consensus when the decision is not healthcare directed by the attending veterinarian. Everyone needs to be allowed to speak his or her mind before the final decision is made. Good leaders ensure that this happens with regularity. Once the decision is final, each team member has an obligation to support it fully, in public and within the team. Usually, serving on a practice team means abiding by its decisions, and arriving at those decisions usually means being able to compromise.

A willingness to try something new

Good team members are like the early explorers. They always look for something new, for unknown horizons to test their skills against. The old ways may be quite good and logical, but that does not mean there isn't room for improvement. Times and clients change. Continuous quality improvement needs to be the rule. The best team members keep an open mind and give their best effort willingly when trying the new ideas or programs.

The ability to see things clearly and to solve problems easily

Often teams are assembled without any attention to fit. In most practices each person is hired for a set of skills, experience, or expertise and thrown into the practice group. When a vexing problem needs to be tackled, one too complicated to be solved by a single individual, identifying the problem in a clear manner is important. This means multiple brains can address the same issue from many perspectives. If a team can accurately define the problem, it is half-solved. Cultivate a balance and neutral problem-solving ability as a team member, and you will be asked for your opinion frequently.

Most likely, those in a veterinary practice have talked about team building. Some practices have accomplished it successfully and others are still trying to find the playing field. Each person was selected to be a member of the healthcare delivery team for a reason, so teamwork must be an expectation of the practice. As good team players, staff members really are trying to build a team to deliver veterinary healthcare to patients that need care. The team members will share some common attributes:

1. Everyone will be committed at the beginning and play hard all the time. No one will sit out on a play and then say "I told you so." People will expose their thoughts and feelings for the team to view and evaluate. It takes courage to be this type of team player.

2. If team members don't know the practice goal or objective, leaders will find a way to define it. They will share this knowledge with others on the team, especially if those others are in the dark.

3. Team members will help determine how to accomplish the practice goals and objectives. They will seek input from others and understand that their own input is important to team success. They will believe that their contribution is just as important to the team's success as the contributions of others.

4. Each staff member will recognize the good intentions of other team members, and each person will state the good that he or she has perceived before discussing how to do things better next time. Team players will downplay their independence for the sake of team intra-dependence, they will respect the skill and expertise of others, and they will freely respect other members of the team.

5. Decision making is a team effort that requires a volunteer on some occasions. A veterinary extender is someone who sees a need and finds a way to meet it without causing extra work for the doctor.

6. Teams will share the success and not backpedal in the light of failure; they will share credit for good ideas that have worked. A good team shares the glory with each other, but a great team celebrates the success of others.

The goals and objectives of the veterinary practice are the methods of scoring, and the technical manual, job descriptions, and employee manual are the rule books for the game. The ability of a veterinary practice to share these items in a clear and concise manner is a critical element of team building. How they are shared sets the tone for team play. In many flourishing practices, job descriptions have been replaced by the authority to solve problems within established guidelines, instead of by the rule book.

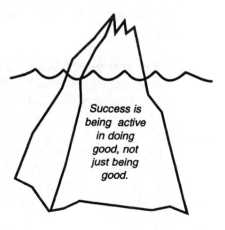

Success is being active in doing good, not just being good.

Personal Roles in the Team

Anyone may become a team star, but even the best stars never forget how they became known. Joe Montana reminded everyone again, at the end of his last season, that he is good because of the other 10 team members on the field. A pass can't be caught by the thrower, a hand-off requires someone else to run, and even a quarterback sneak takes a lot of blocking by the line. Always remember that it is the team score that is entered into the record book, that the team wins the trophy, and every member of the team gets a Super Bowl ring.

In veterinary healthcare the individual members of the team make the client aware of the quality care, deliver concerned care to the pet, and make the practice a nice place to be for staff, clients, and veterinarians. It isn't easy to be a great team player.

In summary, the qualities of a good team player are:

- A willingness to sacrifice for the benefit of the team
- A willingness to let the team leader lead
- The ability to contribute your best as a team member
- A spirit of compromise
- A willingness to try something new
- The ability to see things clearly and to solve problems easily

Listening Skills

The six qualities just mentioned assume one thing: that each team member has developed good listening skills. Listening requires effort, and in most practices, this does not occur. The conversation goes something like this:

"Do you have trouble hearing?" asked the doctor of a new receptionist who sat at her station. "No, Doc," replied the receptionist. "I have trouble listening, just like you."

Decisions are often made in secret by practice owners (not leaders), and the inactivity of the staff is an outward manifestation of the doctor's assumption that everyone will understand intuitively why things are the way they are. We consult with practices whose leaders say they want a team, and we get them to delegate, but the boss never listens to the staff members, or worse, allows the staff members to see only the tips of icebergs and are not trusting enough to let them hear the rest of the story. Funny thing—most Americans are like this: independent and private. They hear, but they don't listen. The ability to listen is not an inborn trait. It takes a conscious effort to do it well. Successful team members are listeners first. And listeners are people who:

Listen Intently

Their minds do not wander. They concentrate on what the other person is saying.

Repress Their Own Egos

They do not interrupt, nor are they formulating a response. They concentrate on the feelings being conveyed and try to understand that the other person is speaking out because he or she cares about the practice.

Are Patient

Nothing is more annoying than a person who has no patience to hear you out. They interrupt and redefine the issues being discussed rather than address the problems from the perspective of the team member speaking.

Are Concerned

They care about what the other person is saying because they care about the person. The desire for team harmony and cooperation is more important than the secrets of the practice business.

In summary, a good listener exhibits these behaviors:

- Listens intently
- Represses own ego
- Is patient
- Is concerned

Listening Feedback Techniques

No one is perfect. We all have some bad listening habits that we get away with when we talk to our family or friends. In a practice

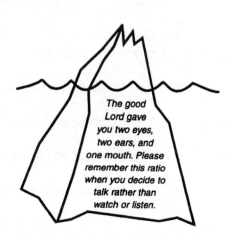

The good Lord gave you two eyes, two ears, and one mouth. Please remember this ratio when you decide to talk rather than watch or listen.

context, however, every team member must leave these bad habits behind and practice active listening. To give you some insight into your own listening habits, a list of common irritating listening habits is provided here. Read through the list and be honest with yourself. Awareness must come before you can start to eliminate these bad habits.

1. You do all the talking—you try to speak louder than the other person.

2. You interrupt another person's train of thought or talk.

3. You do not stop what you are doing to look at the person speaking to you.

4. You continually toy with a pencil, pen, or some other item while talking.

5. Your poker face keeps people guessing whether you understand them.

6. Because you never smile, you come off as too serious.

7. You change what others say by putting your words in their mouth.

8. You put people on the defensive when targeting your questions.

9. You ask questions about what has just been said, showing you weren't listening.

10. You start to debate or argue before the other person is finished talking.

11. Everything said leads to your thinking of an experience you must share immediately.

12. You finish sentences for people if they pause too long.

13. You become angry when someone finishes a sentence for you.

14. You work so hard at eye contact that people become uncomfortable.

15. You evaluate the appearance of the person before listening to him or her.

16. You measure other people's words as believable or unbelievable.

17. Your body language speaks so loudly that the other person is out-shouted.

18. You act as if you know it all, frequently relating savior incidents.

19. You become distracted by thoughts or words and miss the rest of the message.

20. You listen to the words rather than the feelings being shared.

After Listening

Effective listening goes beyond hearing the words that are being said. In fact, less than 25 percent of communication comes from words. Over half is conveyed by body language and over a quarter by vocal tones. Here are some supplemental ideas to consider when trying to improve client (or staff) communications:

Define the words

Try to understand exactly what the client is saying, and use words the client will understand when responding. Most clients are intimidated by the —ology, —otomy, —ectomy, —itis, and other Greek and Latin terminology we use, not to mention the abbreviations, acronyms, jargon, and slang.

In lieu of assumptions

Before acting on an assumption, test it. This is known as active listening, to be sure you understood the person's message. It is okay to ask the client what was really meant, what was really felt, or what he or she really thinks can be done to make it right. It is never wrong to ask another caring and concerned question for clarity.

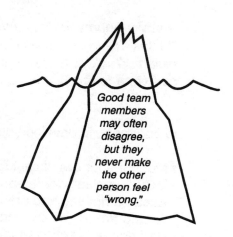

Good team members may often disagree, but they never make the other person feel "wrong."

Create transitions

When you have summed up an issue, ask the client to explain the next issue of concern. This causes the discussion to move onto another facet that needs resolution.

Give nonverbal hints

Use your body language to make the client feel comfortable with your level of concern. Nod your head, face your client squarely, maintain good eye contact, lean slightly forward, withhold reaction or judgments to statements, and remember, smiles work on almost everyone in the United States of America.

Changes Count

A client judges feedback by responsive behavior and by someone in the practice taking action to allay the client's concerns. When you ask, "What is needed to make it right?" the answer must be acted upon within 24 hours for the greatest impact.

Convert to a Question

When a statement is difficult to respond to, ask a question that has a reply you are ready for. For example:

"I don't think I need to buy that product." Your response could be, *"What was the doctor's reason for prescribing this product?"*

"Your price is too high." Respond with a question such as, *"Do you know we take credit cards?"* or *"Do you know that you could spread this cost out by writing multiple checks? Or we could run multiple card imprints, then deposit them over time?"*

"I never approved this service." This one needs a quick reply, such as, *"I think this needs to be discussed with the admitting veterinarian/technician. Would you like to join me in examination room 3, and I will find someone to rectify this issue?"*

In summary, to develop your listening skills:

• Monitor your own listening habits and eliminate the bad ones.
• Define unclear words and terminology.
• Assume nothing and practice active listening.
• Create transitions into other topics of concern.
• Use nonverbal cues (body language) to show that you are listening.

- Practice responsive behavior that reassures the client you have listened.
- Learn to convert a statement for which you have no response into a follow-up question for which you do have a response.

How to Build a Team

If you are a good team player—if you really try to build a team to deliver veterinary healthcare to patients that need your skills—then you will almost certainly possess the attributes we discussed on pages 19–20.

In a veterinary practice, however, the team analogy must go beyond that of the sports arena. An athlete can go to the dressing room at halftime or after a hard-played four-hour game and recuperate. It is not that way in practice. The team is in the center of the action for hours on end, until patient demands and client needs wane.

In team sports, conditioning is both physical and mental, within the expected demands of the sport. The limitations placed on the opponents are well defined, allowing the team to concentrate on their own weaknesses. In veterinary medicine, disease occurrence and bodily injury have no limitations; mutations occur as well as accidents. There is no time-out or instant replay. The conditioning is mental and physical, but the unexpected is the usual.

In a veterinary practice the veterinarian is the quarterback, the coach, the manager, and, during many night emergencies, often the rest of the team. When staff members assume the role of paraprofessional veterinary extenders, they commit to a life of dynamic change ... to excitement based on the unknown and unpredictable ... to a set of rules that are changed by every client encounter and every patient healthcare situation. The requirement to think for oneself is far more important in a healthcare situation.

There is a team synergy that exists in healthcare delivery, and it makes the support of patient needs come naturally. The empathy felt toward team members in times of stress is usually translated into helping hands as well as moral support. The stressed client is not a spectator, but rather another human who needs the team care and concern. A great team player learns to see the healthcare services being offered through the eyes of the client. When the client perceives a greater practice quality

Perceptions start as a mirror of your values— empathy, questions, and factual integration provide better clarity.

because of a staff member's efforts, then successful team play is achieved.

The veterinary practice system of the 1990s demands that the professional and paraprofessional staff grow beyond the sport teams we learned about as kids and enter a greater commitment based on trust and caring, skill and competency, sacrifice and personal tenacity. It does not require a playbook, an umpire, or a sideline coach. A veterinary practice requires total commitment to the profession of veterinary medicine, and not just a few hours at a time. It demands a specialized healthcare delivery team that is able to establish a set of common values to guide their decisions and actions. It also requires a leadership team. Every team member needs to make it his or her challenge to contribute to these practice, staff, and client needs.

In the process of building a team, staff members need to recognize the following:

• There is no time out or time off until the patient's needs are met.
• There are no time clocks, and you must expect the unexpected.
• In the healthcare delivery process, the veterinarian often plays quarterback, coach, manager, and, in some emergencies, the whole team.
• Look at the practice through the client's eyes.
• Look beyond sports analogies as you develop your practice team.

The Infinity Model

I can't get a handle on this management stuff; it just doesn't seem to work

in my practice unless I reduce my personal client contact time.

—Dr. ABC, XY Animal Clinic

For veterinary practices to excel in the 1990s, the principles of management (business basics) must be married to the integrative concepts of leadership. The basic premise of any leadership situation is that there are followers. The M.B.A.-like training model pursued by some veterinary managers excludes the followers, thereby negating the healthcare delivery team concept. The veterinary practice owner deserves the chance to include a paraprofessional in a management training program and see team training in an interactive problem-based environment.

The infinity model for veterinary practice success in the future basically combines the two concepts of leadership and business in a single flow diagram, as in Figure 1.1.

I call this integrated concept an "infinity model" because it is a process,

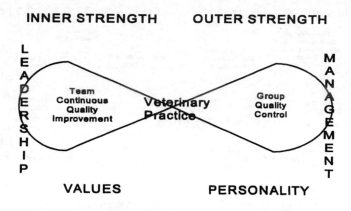

INNER STRENGTH   OUTER STRENGTH

VALUES   PERSONALITY

Fig. 1.1. Basic dynamic system veterinary practice model

not a program. It is a mind-set and a commitment to excellence that empowers the team, makes every individual accountable to develop a better tomorrow, and stays centered on the goal of quality healthcare delivery. Although there must be total commitment by the leader for the model to have a beginning, it has no end. It is an infinity model because the goal is to exceed expectations, thus instilling pride within the individual. Once goals are exceeded, new objectives need to be jointly set so a higher level of productivity, performance, and pride can be achieved.

Personal growth needs to be supported and promoted on a continual basis for each team member, not just for the M.B.A.-like leaders. When the input is pride in performance, the output is the perception of quality by the client. The client's perception of quality is the true measurement of successful healthcare delivery in a client-centered environment. The infinity model is just the beginning of the basic components for team training ideas.

Schools of Thought

The right side of the advanced infinity model (see Figure 1.2) shows the basic concerns and cornerstones of business—the veterinary management programs of the 1980s. The left side of the model reflects the basic skills and principles associated with leadership—the veterinary management programs evolving in the 1990s. Neither side can be used in isolation, nor

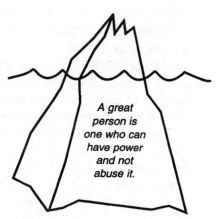

A great person is one who can have power and not abuse it.

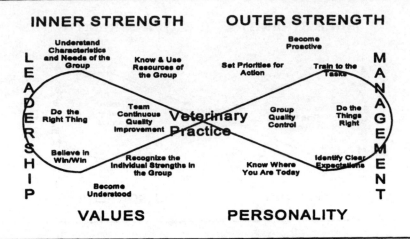

Fig. 1.2. Advanced dynamic system veterinary practice model

can it be learned in isolation. Leaders need followers, and those followers are the healthcare team that delivers the care and operates the management functions in a veterinary practice. Although both schools of thought are critical to success, leadership skills cause greater team involvement and easier implementation of the business models.

Veterinarians have always expected their staffs to do the things right. Job descriptions and technical manuals proliferated in the 1980s. But the most successful leaders taught their healthcare teams to do the right things. They were client centered and met the practice's needs rather than just followed the rules.

To progress, you must first know where you are today. That was a basic principle to measure success in the 1980s. In the 1990s we have discovered it is more important to become understood first, to share the dreams, visions, and goals of the practice. Instead of just clearly identifying expectations as we did in the 1980s, we have become concerned with establishing win/win expectations in healthcare team relations.

In the 1980s those who were leading teams learned to set priorities for action, and the jobs got done more efficiently. In the 1990s we have begun to understand people are hired to solve problems rather than just do a job. In the 1980s we stressed training to the tasks, so we would prevent failure. In the 1990s we have learned to educate for the future, so as a healthcare team we can seize opportunities as they arise.

The leadership skills for the 1990s are based on recognizing the individual strengths and resources within the group combined with understanding the characteristics and needs of the individual and group. The management skills of the 1980s were based on becoming proactive.

The skill of sharing leadership has never been considered essential in management, which is why delegation was often ineffective. Assigning accountabilities (1990s) requires independent decisions and continual progress, while delegation (1980s) means employees do the assigned job without supervision. This simple concept is critical to the difference between the quality control programs of the 1980s and the continuous quality improvement efforts of the 1990s.

These schools of thought are combined in the infinity model because all the concepts are essential to developing a comprehensive management model for veterinary practice performance and productivity in the future. Values and inner strength are critical binding elements for leadership skills, whereas personality and outer strengths are the binding agents that enable business management skills to take shape. The skills of planning and evaluating cross the boundaries of management and leadership, but the skill of controlling the group changes from didactic styles to participative styles when accepting the importance of leadership in veterinary practice management.

Teaching Versus Learning

We all experienced different kinds of teachers as we grew up and made our life choices, but the true educators were those who cared if we were learning. There are teachers who would disagree with this simplistic example, but think back to those who have most affected your life. Did they stand in front and talk at you, or did they live the example they wanted you to set and go the extra mile to ensure you understood why?

The healthcare team can be *taught* the tasks and functions on the right side of the model, or they can *learn* to use their strengths to solve the problems associated with the business of veterinary practice. Nothing kills creative and innovative juices like being trained to the tasks. Our patients are trained, but people learn to train. The way we treat our staff members reflects the methods they will use to deal with our clients. Educated clients come to the healthcare team for assistance more often than trained clients. The genius of leadership is to educate others and to create situations that allow team members to solve problems so they believe they can do so without the leader.

The most effective management courses of the 1990s will be the problem-based learning experiences, whether it be in medicine or management skills. The secret of management is that it requires a team ef-

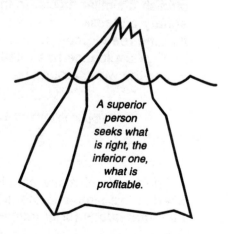

A superior
person
seeks what
is right, the
inferior one,
what is
profitable.

fort, because it does not produce income in itself. Management involves people, and people respond to leaders, whether their names be Lincoln, Churchill, or Disney, or if they just go by letters, like JFK or Dr. ABC.

We need to educate leaders, and we need to educate the healthcare team. We can do so in isolation, or we can support each other centrally, at the community or state veterinary medical association (VMA) level. As long as we promote segregation of continuing education between the leaders and the followers, teams will harbor their own expectations. Management needs to be an integrated process, wherein the professionals and paraprofessionals share a learning experience, develop personal skills, then come back together to integrate the skills to a higher level of performance, productivity, and profitability. When pride becomes the input of all parties, then quality will be the outcome perceived by the client. When the client perceives quality in service, then the price will be worth the value.

Which part of the infinity model have you been developing in your practice? Have you gotten the results you wanted? Can the progress be quicker, more effective, or more fun? Are you willing to make the adjustments and commitment to accept a new process that does not have an end? Continuous quality improvement is a new lifestyle within healthcare delivery, and the principles do carry over into personal lifestyles. Are you ready to meet the emerging needs of the 1990s?

The Values of Granddad

The May 6, 1991, issue of *Time* magazine had a great cover article, about the Cult of Greed. Owning a business devoted to full-time veterinary practice management consulting, I had to stop and reflect on our profession. No journal or magazine in our profession has had the courage to publish a similar article. In fact, most of the recent articles about the veterinary profession, or about its management arm, have been so guarded that the reader may have a hard time telling what the intent of the article is. Risk avoidance has ruled our profession for years, but it has also affected the world around us.

> *If you don't stand for something, you will fall for anything.*
> —Granddad

The words of many people come to mind here, and they are summarized in this simple quote. It seems that most people enjoy talking about their granddads (or grandmas) and the values they had, which can make us stop and think about the roots of this country. As I reviewed theories of practice management during my M.H.A. studies at Baylor University, I could easily see that the history of styles of management changed following World War I. The grandparents we all cherish formed their values in those times before World War I, the times when inner strength had priority over image.

During the first 150 years of this country, our leaders had values. A handshake meant something, a person's word was his or her bond. I don't know if the change occurred during the industrial revolution, the market crash, the urbanization of America, or a phase of the moon, but our national values are certainly not what they once were. Before World War I the U.S.A. had a rural-based lifestyle, what we call conservative today. People helped their neighbors without being asked, they didn't sue just because an accident occurred, and, more important, they believed in hard work, not a quick fix.

> *In matters of style, swim with the current;*
> *in matters of principle, stand like a rock.*
> —*Thomas Jefferson*

The reason for this values dilemma isn't our profession's fault. Since World War I the entire U.S.A. work ethic has evolved to a me-based or immediate gratification philosophy. People who work hard are ridiculed, usually by those risk avoiders who want to maintain the status quo. Innovative or creative people are usually termed mavericks, or even boat rockers. In the late 1970s Congress had to enact legislation to protect those who reported waste and fraud in government (whistle blowers). Compare these events to the stories of granddad and grandma; their stories are filled with hard work, personal ethics, and life values that anyone can admire, especially those who claim they are related to people with those kinds of inner strengths.

Our profession hasn't had many choices when it comes to veterinary practice consultants. The ethical professionals available within our profession are usually in one-person consulting services that don't promise the moon without looking at your practice. The reputable multipeople systems are not veterinary specific or trained, and the ones like those *Time* featured will generally promise you anything for reasons not usually germane to the practice philosophy.

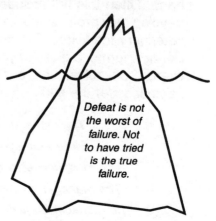

Defeat is not the worst of failure. Not to have tried is the true failure.

The quest for a veterinary medical degree takes many years; profession-ally, we understand that a femoral head resection comes at the end of a long quest for knowledge, because we must understand the physics, anatomy, and physiological impact of the procedure to be competent. In the search for the easy way to manage, we forget that learning the basics is a requirement for a professional understanding of why something needs to be done. Learning the theory and concepts allows independent replica-tion at a later date.

If you were to sell your character, would you get full retail,

or would it go for a bargain-basement price with discount coupons?

—Grandma

The ethical and professional consultants have spent many years build-ing their skills, and it hasn't come easy for them. The study of veterinary practice management should be built on experience, study, education, or a combination of all these factors. This depth of knowledge leads to an un-derstanding that individuals are different, practices are different, and one answer doesn't fit all. The reputable consultants respect the individual and do not base assistance on the depth of credit line available. They know when to network with other experts in the field of veterinary medical prac-tice management, or when to stop an engagement because they can no longer help the practice or veterinarian; individual personalities and differ-ences are respected.

When the current techniques of practice management consulting are evaluated, they usually fall into the categories of leadership or manage-ment. The leader uses management, whereas the manager uses pro-grams and gimmicks. A good practice consultant will find the cause and effect of existing problems and build on the strengths of the resources at hand. Often this will include recommending that the veterinarian or staff develop new professional skills and confidences, in both management and veterinary medicine. The manager-based consultant looks only at things like new forms, a glossier yellow-page ad, a newspaper campaign to steal clients from colleagues, or new sales tricks and arbitrary performance ex-pectations for the staff.

The manager administers, the leader innovates.

The manager maintains, the leader develops.

The manager relies on systems, the leader relies on people.

The manager counts on controls, the leader counts on trust.

The manager does things right, the leader does the right things.

—Fortune Magazine

As I see it, the difference between a leader and a manager is often a difference of values and inner strength. We must believe in a leader to follow, but we only need to follow a program if a manager's in charge. The current literature on management usually emphasizes a search for traits that people can follow. The American management scene was founded on the ethics and values of our grandparents, but we are now being sold on the quick fix, assigning the blame, finding the easy way or the oversimplified approach of slick promotion and glib promises that are expected to be broken.

Some practice management techniques are based on leadership, but most written about today are based on management. Mind control is a method of management; empowerment is a method of leadership—but it is a belief, not a technique. Assigning tasks and measurements are manager aides; assigning accountabilities marks the leader. If you are considering obtaining the services of a veterinary practice consultant, look for the values that are founded on our grandparents' values. The veterinary practice team is a family, and the same values and inner strengths are required to achieve feelings of accomplishment and personal harmony. Arriving at this family team concept is as easy as growing up, and that was a long-term challenge for everyone.

Building a management team is also a long-term commitment. To achieve continuous quality improvement in a practice, pride must be a common value of every staff member. This ideal requires a group of people who will put personal agendas aside and build on the practice dream. Not everyone will have the work ethic or values of our grandparents, especially at the wages veterinary practices pay. Although you can't control an individual's attitude, you can expect behavior to meet the practice's needs. How we elicit this behavior is reflected in the "dynamic system" diagram and the manager versus leader discussion in this book.

The infinity diagram depicts a few of the choices and key techniques available to the practice owner. Either route can make a practice successful, and energies of management can flow easily in both directions. In fact, the balance between the two sides of the dynamic system is sometimes critical to success. There are some of us, though, who cannot equate financial success with personal success; this success concept is often one of the underlying causes for professional burnout. As you review the infinity diagram, think about where you want to be in five years, not tomorrow. It takes time to change and even longer to

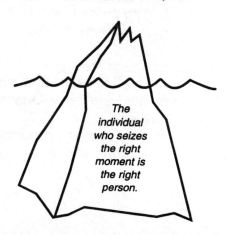

The individual who seizes the right moment is the right person.

change the practice habits of a lifetime. Compare the alternative routes to the practice management styles of the consultants who interest you; look to the end result that you really want, including quality of life; and remember the following idea that I got from my granddad:

All people have a choice in life;
they may approach it as
creator or critic,
builder or watcher,
lover or hater,
giver or taker.

■ ■ ■ Review ■ ■ ■

In this chapter we covered information that defines what a team player is, how to be a team player, how to develop good listening skills, and how to start building a team. From these basic concepts we can go on to define and develop personal leadership skills. Be sure you understand the information in this lesson before you continue to Chapter 2: The Framework.

1. A team player possesses:
    a. A willingness to sacrifice for the benefit of the team
    b. A willingness to let leaders lead
    c. A willingness to contribute one's best to the team
    d. A spirit of compromise
    e. A willingness to risk new adventures
    f. The ability to see facts without bias
    g. A willingness to solve problems

2. Listening means:
    a. Hearing words and understanding why
    b. Studying body language and voice tone to understand what is meant
    c. Being patient, concerned, and open-minded
    d. Hearing all of the message before formulating a response

3. Attributes of a good team player are:
   a. Total commitment
   b. Finding ways to define goals or objectives with other team members
   c. Helping to accomplish goals and objectives
   d. Seeing the good intentions of other team members
   e. A willingness to volunteer for projects based on group decision, without causing extra work for others
   f. Sharing successes and forging ahead in the event of failure

CHAPTER TWO

The Framework

Skills of Leadership

*When it is all said and done, there are but two objectives of
veterinary practice leadership: (1) accomplish the practice mission, and
(2) ensure the welfare of the people on the team.*
—Dr. T. E. Cat

Definition of Leadership

Leadership is the difference between average and excellent practice
management. Leadership is the art of influencing and directing others in
such a way as to obtain their confidence, respect, and loyal cooperation in
order to accomplish the mission of the veterinary practice.

Some practice owners confuse the veterinary healthcare delivery mission with their own personal beliefs and bias about ancillary functions, but
this is not the stuff of which leaders are made. The simplest check is to
look at the following indicators of leadership within a specific veterinary
practice:

Morale
The state of mind of the individual. This state of mind is dependent upon
the person's attitudes toward everything that affects him or her in the
practice sphere of influence. It is reality, regardless of the perceptions of
the practice's owner, and it mirrors the environment established by the
leadership.

Discipline
The prompt observance of protocols and policies and, in the absence of
additional doctor orders, the initiation of appropriate action for the welfare of the client, patient, and practice. A form of self-direction and personal accountability for improved outcomes.

Esprit de Corps
The *loyalty to*, the *pride in*, and the *enthusiasm for* the practice and what it stands for, as shown by the staff to clients, the doctor, each other, and the community.

Proficiency
The technical knowledge and skill, as well as the professional attitude and physical ability, to do a job well. Proficiency is the ability to accomplish the practice mission without immediate direction and supervision; it is excellence.

The leadership of any practice should hire for attitude and train for skills when building a healthcare delivery team. Those unwilling to join the team should be released to find a group or environment that better fits their level of commitment and attitude. The following are signs of management fatigue and leadership neglect:

- If you can't trust someone to do _____, there is an indication of poor leadership development within the team.
- If someone has a bad attitude, there is an indication of poor leadership development within the team.
- If someone does not have the pride and enthusiasm to contribute to new practice programs, there is an indication of poor leadership development within the team.
- If someone cannot be trusted to wear the proper dress, or maintain an orderly work space, there is an indication of poor leadership development within the team.

Traits of Leadership

A leadership trait or characteristic is a quality of personality. In sum, these qualities of personality are of greatest assistance in obtaining confidence, respect, and loyal cooperation by those within their sphere of influence. There are a dozen *essential leadership traits* for those building a veterinary healthcare delivery team:

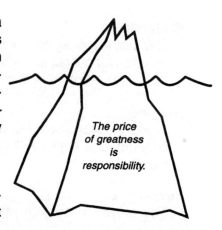

The price of greatness is responsibility.

Integrity
Consistency and soundness of moral principle, absolute truthfulness and honesty at

each turn of a practice day, and the ability to be trusted, in word and action, in practice operations.

Knowledge
Acquired information put into practical application in quality veterinary healthcare delivery; an understanding of the right thing for the right reason, and at the right time.

Courage
The mental quality that recognizes fear (of danger or criticism) but enables a leader to proceed in the face of adversity with calmness, predictable values, and firmness.

Decisiveness
An ability to reach decisions promptly and to announce them in a clear and concise manner; the certainty of the proper performance by the veterinarian's oath and bioethical principles.

Initiative
Seeing what has to be done and commencing a course of action, even in the absence of directions; ensuring an opportunity is not lost to enhance the practice or the welfare of a client or patient.

Confidence
Conveying an image of self-worth, and protecting the self-worth of others; accepting the blame for others as a personal training shortfall, thereby developing better programs for the future.

Tact
The ability to deal with others without creating offense, enhanced by the quality of being impartial and consistent in exercising leadership judgment.

Enthusiasm
The display of sincere interest and exuberance in the performance of practice functions, including the positive aspects of anyone's ideas and the positive potential in even the most adverse of conditions.

Bearing
Creating a favorable impression in carriage, appearance, and personal conduct at all times, within the practice setting as well as within the community.

Judgment
The quality of weighing facts and factors against possible alternatives,

in harmony with team members; establishing a sound basis for decisions that may impact upon others.

Loyalty
Faithfulness to the practice values and the veterinary medical profession; dependability and concern for the feelings of others on the team.

Selflessness
Avoidance of providing for one's own comfort and personal advancement at the expense of others; weighing the needs of self against the needs of the practice, doctors, staff, clients, and patients.

These dozen essential traits are implemented in different manners in different practices, often by exception, and more often as isolated actions not integrated into the total practice philosophy. In fact, most practices never establish an integrated program of staff development and leadership expectations. The development of a program is most often left to chance. Leadership is an art as well as a science. Knowing the traits and having the ability to list the principles does not make for a great leader. Being able to speak the words is still the student's approach. The true leader exhibits these traits in an unconscious manner in each action of each day.

When a leader performs within a practice setting, the outward signs of leadership are often perceived as practice principles. The attitudes associated with these principles cause the aforementioned indicators of leadership to emerge. There are a dozen principles of action that reflect the traits of leadership:

1. Be technically proficient, and train others to be proficient.

2. Know yourself and seek self-improvement regularly.

3. Support your staff and look out for their welfare.

4. Keep the team members informed and striving for improvement.

5. Be consistent and set the example at all times.

6. Ensure that the task is understood, supervised, and accomplished.

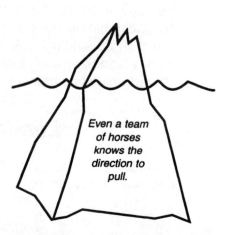

Even a team of horses knows the direction to pull.

7. Train the staff members as a competent team.

8. Make sound and timely decisions, in healthcare and staff management.

9. Develop a sense of responsibility among the team members, and recognize effort.

10. Assign projects in accordance with the capabilities of the individual.

11. Seek responsibility and take accountability for outcomes and actions.

12. Expect excellence, pursue continuous improvement, and celebrate the attempt.

Ideally, actions of the practice owners should be guided by the traits and principles of leadership—but that would be utopia. Leadership techniques exhibit the traits and apply the principles, but no one can be all things to all people. Leadership is a never-ending struggle to excel, and to remain consistent in the eyes of the other staff members. The good news is that winning the struggle usually causes increased staff tenure and practice excellence, unless the leader loses his or her vision and reverts to a merely managerial role.

The impact of a crashing management program is most often seen in a high turnover rate among the staff. A disenchanted staff is not a happy staff, and veterinary practices seldom pay enough for people to stay unhappy and keep coming to work. They will depart the practice. So if you plan to embark on a leadership development program in your practice and accept accountability for continuous improvement, also accept the fact that sound leadership is a forever process, not a start and stop program. Be ready to accept the stress of developing others while sacrificing self, of accepting blame and giving credit, and of doing the right things instead of just doing things right. A successful practice leader evolves into a community leader, so don't ever believe the quest will be over. Once you have started, the world needs you. Never give up!

Leadership Principles

Let's put the two terms "management" and "leadership" into a perspective that we can easily understand.

❑ Managers focus on the near-term tasks and activities.
■ Leaders stress promotion of long-term team effectiveness.

❑ Managers take credit and give blame.
■ Leaders give credit and take blame.

❑ You can lead a horse to water ... but ...
■ You can't manage a horse to water ...

❑ You can manage a project or staff, or do it yourself.
■ Leaders must have followers, or they can't be leaders.

Burt Nanus, coauthor of *Leaders: The Strategies for Taking Charge*, says that to become a leader you need to develop certain vital qualities and skills. As seen in many practices visited, the following qualities become essential for success:

Farsightedness
Understand the future.
Learn from the past.
Assess the human resources available.
Check the long-term trends.
Develop a realistic vision.
Promote staff enthusiasm.
Have a common team goal.

Flexibility
Adapt your goals to changing conditions.
Control surprises.
Monitor performance against goals.
Make decisions promptly.
Set firm deadlines.
Speed the tempo of the group.

Managing by Design
Continually shape the group.
Use productivity instruments.
Discuss job descriptions thoroughly.
Issue clear policy statements.
Initiate a program of staff training.
Encourage shared identity among staff.

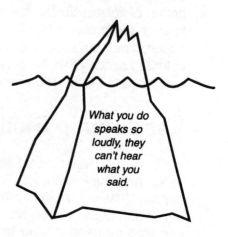

What you do speaks so loudly, they can't hear what you said.

Continuous Learning
Widen your horizons.
Read the trade journals.
Attend seminars.
Network with success.
Unlearn obsolete ways.

Integrity
Win staff trust.
Make only promises that can be kept.
Trust your team.
Share goals and work plans.
Give staff decision-making authority.

To the traditional student of veterinary practice management, life is a series of gimmicks (not a box of chocolates, as stated by Forrest Gump). Most traditional veterinarians want guarantees for every new idea they try and many of them want others to change so they can stay the same; these are not the traits of a true leader. The five qualities listed above are not common in most practice owners; the practice schedule is often perceived as too demanding to do "all of this leadership stuff." The problem is, the traits of the group must also be the traits of the leadership, and what is actually done by the leadership speaks so loudly the staff cannot hear what is being said. A skill can be learned and a trait exhibited, so leadership may be seen by some veterinary professionals as applied skills, but it goes beyond that level of learning the gimmicks. There is a caring which precedes a team formation, and it is the concern the leader shows for the feelings and value of each team member which is the foundation of this caring. We have developed a series of fourteen skills which are the foundation of successful leadership and the first three are specifically designed to form the group, while the next two are transitional skills of group interaction. The balance of the skills are used by both the groups and the individual to accomplish the tasks at hand and the challenges of the future, as well as help the practice evolve within the community support.

Leadership Skills for Veterinary Practices

There are some basic leadership skills which have been taught for years and they remain as important today as they did at the turn of the century. These historical skills have been used to develop and integrated set of operational leadership skills for veterinary practices. These 14 skills can also be used in your family, any workplace, a volunteer organization of your choice, and even your church group. Consider the following sequence of leadership skills:

■ Knowing and using the resources of the group

■ Understanding the characteristics and needs of the group

■ Effective communications

■ Reflection

■ Representing the group

■ Evaluating

■ Effective teaching

■ Planning

■ Internal promotion

■ Situational leadership

■ Group development

■ Personal relationships

■ Setting the example

■ Continuous quality improvement (CQI)

Let's look at each skill individually:

Knowing and using the resources of the group means you depend on what members of the team can do, as well as on what you can do. To use these resources, you must first know what they are. Watch the members in action, talk to them over lunch, watch for abilities and interest areas. You will know when you are using the resources of the group when others begin to lead and the practice programs are more than just the result of your ideas.

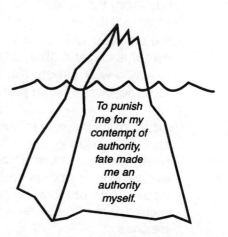

To punish me for my contempt of authority, fate made me an authority myself.

Understanding the group's characteristics and needs means that everyone on the staff, including the leaders, remembers that each staff member comes from a different background. Each person has strengths and weaknesses that affect the practice team and the harmony within. Some call this skill "learning the hot buttons," but it goes further than that; it is caring enough to lend a hand because you know there is a need. By understanding each team member's individual needs, everyone benefits.

Effective communication occurs when, despite a world overloaded with data from the media and from computers, you can both get and give information (defined as raw data that has been processed by some logical or caring person) effectively and efficiently. Taking notes is one method that illustrates you are effectively processing information, asking questions shows that data has been converted to information, and getting feedback means that the message you sent was received. Discuss things that are going to happen in the practice. In healthcare you measure your success in terms of getting the job done and the degree to which instructions are followed.

Reflecting is balancing the characteristics and needs of the individual with the needs of the group. It is a transitional skill between forming the group (first three skills) and getting the group to work in harmony to achieve a specific task, objective, or milestone. Reflecting is what a caring leader does to balance the stresses and mission needs with the people needs of his team.

Representing the group can be seen from the viewpoint of either the leadership or the staff. Sometimes even the clients get a spokesperson among the staff. The staff represent the values of the veterinarian every day, from the receptionist to the technician. The ideas and suggestions of the staff flow through middle managers to the practice's owner, and the practice policies and procedures come from the professional and owner level through middle managers back to the staff. Representation is a two-way street. You are succeeding in this area when everyone feels he or she has a part in the practice's decisions and operation.

Evaluating is more than keeping a scorecard. Everyone assesses a situation both during and after the event. For the evaluation process to work, you must have a goal for each activity. A set of expectations that everyone can understand is the measuring standard before an event occurs. The practice philosophy, its core values, and the mission statement are the guidelines that should form expectations of the evaluation process.

Effective teaching is more than talking at people. Don't assume the staff have learned something just because you've written a protocol manual or taught it once. The proof lies in what they can do. The trick is to put them in a position where they see the need for the skill or knowledge you wish them to learn, then offer help. After they think they have learned the skill, let them try it themselves, monitored by someone who knows what the predetermined standards are for the practice. Replication is learning; improvement is knowledge.

Planning lies at the core of a successful veterinary practice. A leader must plan when no one else can, but good leaders don't do the planning for the team for very long. As soon as possible, train your team to do the planning. When the staff assume the responsibility for the planning process, they also assume the operational activities of daily practice. When the team is doing its job, healthcare delivery becomes fun again.

Internal promotion is based on the premise that clients are more than customers. They have a social contract with the practice to provide peace of mind concerning their animal. As clients they can be led and should be educated to enhance their decisions. They need to be allowed to buy from more than one alternative. They should never feel they have been sold something. A leader in veterinary medicine will also be a community leader, and this leadership will enhance practice success.

Situational leadership means tailoring one's approach to the team and to the situation at hand. In health or safety issues the veterinarian must be very *direct* and *instructional*. With new staff, *persuasion* and *coaching* must frequently be used to enhance confidence. *Delegating* means to release control of the process but requires very clear expectations of outcome (which become the leadership control). Once a program has been delegated, the leader becomes a *consultant* and doesn't take it back—ever! The most participative style of leadership is *joining the group*, as with parties or other social events. No one style is ever appropriate all the time.

Group development is based on the premise that any group is a dynamic entity, with its own ebb and flow. People enter the group with high hopes and a positive attitude. New people need to find their niche in the group and in the practice, which can

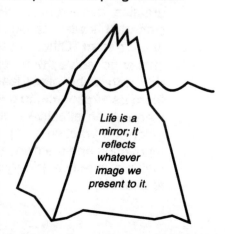

Life is a mirror; it reflects whatever image we present to it.

be stressful. Tenured staff must release turf to new staff or new programs, which can also cause stress and frustration. The skilled leader accelerates the normalization of the group and sets clear expectations for performance. The team in harmony will exceed expectations and reach beyond the routine. The cycle repeats itself with additions of new people, programs, or stresses. The skilled leader guides the group to new levels of excellence.

Personal relationships is a simple phrase, but an integrative process. It requires the skilled leader to go more than halfway in any relationship. When people are willing to go only halfway, there remains a middle barrier. When someone is willing to do what it takes, the barriers that derail good personal relationships disappear. A caring leader makes the barriers disappear for all the people in the group.

The example you set—what you do—speaks louder than anything you can ever say. How you treat your staff is the same way the staff will treat your clients. Set the example of caring at all times for clients, staff, and their families. Everything you do sets the tone for your staff: how you speak to them and treat them, the ways you interact with the community, your pursuit of continuing education. The manner in which you present yourself to clients and staff, physically and emotionally, will establish how the practice as a whole presents itself. The way you act should be in harmony with the practice philosophy, core values, and mission statement. Double standards have no place in leadership.

Continuous quality improvement involves a commitment to make tomorrow better than today, next week better than last week, next month better than this month. It is a process embraced by the uncommon leader, given to every staff member in the practice. It centers on improved results for the client, the patient, the staff, and, therefore, the practice. It is a form of empowerment, but extends beyond the task assigned. It is what causes the last item of a traditional job description to change from "Other duties as assigned" to the CQI phrase, "Meet the challenge, solve the problem, make the improvement; just do it!" It carries with it the other leadership skills—from seeing everyone on the team as a resource, to understanding their characteristics and needs, to planning an effective teaching program so the team members can develop the practice group and evaluate the needs of tomorrow. It is the innovation and creativity that make good practices great and change the well-managed veterinary practice into a well-led team of healthcare professionals.

None of the 14 skills can be mastered alone. All require a group to become reality. The group will form into a team when certain operational questions can be answered truthfully and consistently by the leader:

What excites me today?

What can I do today to improve myself?
    ... my practice?
    ... my relationships?

What do I have to be grateful for today?

Who loves me and whom do I love?

What do my clients perceive?

What are our hospital's strengths?

What are the three objectives for today?
    ... this week?
    ... this month?
    ... this quarter?
    ... this year?

These questions lead to discoveries that the 14 leadership skills can impact. The leadership skills can be learned and applied within any veterinary practice. The secret is that each must be applied at the appropriate time for the benefit of the group and the practice. They must be used as a set of true values and operational concepts, not individual quick fixes to meet the crisis of the moment. When used as the 14 tenets that set the leadership tone, they are the foundation of team building, and a team is the strongest force possible in veterinary healthcare delivery.

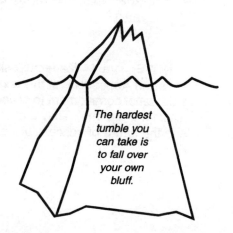

The hardest tumble you can take is to fall over your own bluff.

In summary, you want to be aware of the following and practice them as often as possible with your team:

1. There is a difference between management and leadership:

   a. You don't manage a horse to water, you lead it; as a veterinarian with a stomach tube, you can also make the horse drink.

   b. Require behavior to meet the practice standards.

   c. Attitude is internal to each person and can only be self-motivated.

   d. Leaders change the environment and team members respond.

2. Develop the vital qualities and techniques required for problem solving:
   a. Farsightedness
   b. Flexibility
   c. Managing by design
   d. Continuous learning
   e. Integrity

3. Traits and skills have evolved from different influences experienced by each leader; you are a sum of what has gone before. The other team members are a result of their life experiences and are a sum of what has gone before. Respect this difference.

4. Practice the 14 basic leadership skills:
   a. They should be based on the core values of the practice.
   b. The values are the foundation of all actions and cannot have variable standards in reality or in perception.

5. Monitor the operational CQI questions:
   a. What excites me today?
   b. What can I do today to improve myself, the practice, my relationships?
   c. What do I have to be grateful for today?
   d. What do my clients perceive?
   e. What are our hospital's strengths?
   f. What are the three objectives for today (week, month, quarter, year)?

NOTE: The 14 leadership skills are further explained on one-page summary sheets in Appendix B of this text. The skills are developed over time. They require a personal commitment to action. Don't rush them and don't think they are a gimmick for the month. They are a new way of life, a new way of personal interaction, and the future of successful practices.

Evaluating Your Leadership
Qualities (LQ)

*President Harry Truman once defined leadership as "the ability to get
other people to do what they don't want to do and like it."
To help you determine how good you are at this admittedly
difficult skill, here is a short self-quiz
(select the answer that describes your USUAL approach/effort).*

The following LQ self-evaluation (for practice owners) can be a starting
point. Circle the answers and add up your scores (the number before each
reply).

I trust my staff and make sure they know I believe in them as individuals.
   1. Hardly ever (They know it without my telling them in action or deed.)
   2. Seldom in a month (In general, to the group as a whole, more often.)
   3. Sometimes (At least one person each week, and nearly everybody
      each month.)
   4. Often in a week (Almost every person hears, sees, or feels it weekly.)
   5. Almost daily (I look for ways to reinforce each person, specifically,
      each day.)

**I resist short-term reactions and look toward long-term plans and
goals.**
   1. Hardly ever (If I don't take action, it can hurt the practice.)
   2. Seldom (In general, this is too much effort for most practice activities.)
   3. Sometimes (At least once each month.)
   4. Often (In fact, our annual plan is based on our three-year plan.)
   5. Almost always (Our quarterly plan supports our annual and three-
      year plan.)

**I know how to keep my cool in a crisis and encourage others by my
example.**
   1. Hardly ever (I am known for my temper.)
   2. Seldom (The staff knows which days to avoid my wrath.)
   3. Sometimes (No more than once a month.)
   4. Often (I seldom get pushed into a reaction.)
   5. Almost always (They comment on my positive attitude and total com-
      posure.)

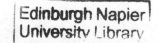

I am a prudent risk taker; I do not refuse to try something different because I fear failure.
1. Hardly ever (I want to be sure of success before we start something new.)
2. Seldom (I need to know the idea has worked elsewhere before we try it.)
3. Sometimes (If they can sell me on the idea, we'll try it.)
4. Often (My efforts are designed to cause creativity and innovation.)
5. Almost always (Continuous improvement/change from each person is required.)

I do my homework and am knowledgeable about all aspects of my practice's business.
1. Hardly ever (I know medicine and surgery, my CPA knows the business.)
2. Seldom (I know the bottom line, others deal with staff issues.)
3. Sometimes (People and progress go together, we talk about it.)
4. Often (I know the income centers, expense centers, and delegation techniques.)
5. Almost always (Accountability for outcomes are based on business planning.)

I invite dissent among my staff and am open to the suggestions they make.
1. Hardly ever (No one rocks the boat in this practice.)
2. Seldom (I know what we need and they have their job descriptions.)
3. Sometimes (People, unrest, and change go together; we talk about it.)
4. Often (I expect to be challenged and give them frequent opportunities.)
5. Almost always (Only those who care dissent; we nurture dissent and new ideas.)

I focus on what's essential and don't get bogged down with useless details.
1. Hardly ever (I need to be involved in the decisions to ensure success.)
2. Seldom (If I don't know what is happening, things often go astray.)
3. Sometimes (In many daily operations others have the decision power.)
4. Often (Once something is delegated, I never take it back or interfere.)
5. Almost always (People are given the accountability for decisions and outcomes.)

I'm an enthusiastic and positive practice manager.
1. Hardly ever
2. Seldom
3. Sometimes
4. Often
5. Almost always

✔ **Over 34 means you are there. Outstanding!**
✔ **A score of 27 to 34 is solid and respectable.**
✔ **A score of 20 to 26 reflects a reliable leader who could get better.**
✔ **Under 20 means you have found a major practice problem, and improvements are necessary.**

Commitment

There are those who speak of "high commitment" for veterinary practice teams. Commitment is fuel for the team. Without it, a team will accomplish very little; with it, there are not many practice limits. Yet commitment has a mysterious quality—it can be there one moment and gone the next. Most often commitment is a by-product of the other components of the 2.1 model; most gimmick-based leaders do not understand this relationship requirement. Note this concept: *Commitment is a by-product of having the practice purpose understood and agreed to by all, having job roles clarified, and ensuring that feedback is working properly.*

Cracking the Nut

It is easy to downplay commitment as a by-product of purpose, job role, and feedback, but they actually interrelate (Figure 2.1). There is a Team TPR (total personal response) evaluation included in this chapter, in case a calibration is desired. We need to define some terms before we proceed much further:

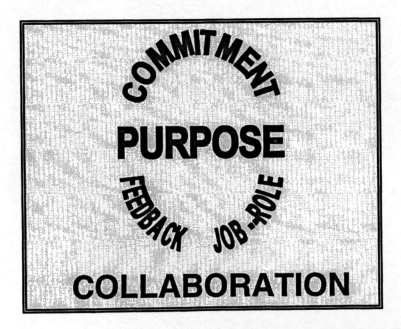

Fig. 2.1. Commitment model

Purpose

The core of the model—its purpose—is central to success; it is most often defined in terms of values, mission, and/or philosophy. This is the hub around which all else evolves. With it a team can be effective; they can grasp why they exist as a team.

Job Role

If the individual's role becomes unclear, confused, or ambiguous, the team becomes ineffective. Although confusion is common during times of change, a leader reduces the stress by offering transitional methods to handle uncertainty and ambiguity.

Feedback

Feedback is absolutely necessary for the team to develop, grow, and prosper. It is what allows each person to know when he or she is approaching the target, how to make corrections required for a bull's-eye, and what adjustments are needed for the next attempt. Feedback is simply the spotlight on those things that are most important to success.

Commitment

The question of commitment within a team is really a question of investment by the individual. Investment dividends are a clear job role and effective feedback, based on meeting the purpose. Commitment is a passion to stay focused, even in the rough times; it is the fuel that keeps things running. It is a sense of both empowerment and personal alignment with the expected outcome. In short, it is coming into line with the team (collaboration).

Collaboration

The foundation of collaboration in the model reflects how a job role is supposed to evolve, how feedback mechanisms are most effective, and even how the practice purpose must forge a common bond between all the team members. Collaboration means working together to make tomorrow better, meeting challenges as they emerge and preventing them from becoming distractions, and most important, always going more than halfway to help another staff member or client when a need is perceived.

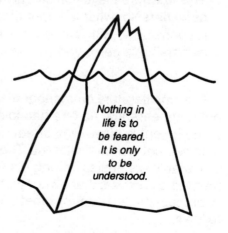

Nothing in life is to be feared. It is only to be understood.

So what does this model mean? In the Jones and Bearley text *Commitment to Vision* (1986), the definition offered states: "Meaningful participation leads to a sense of involvement that evokes a feeling of influence that generates psychological ownership that results in commitment." Think about the components:

Meaningful Participation

Being there isn't enough; "doing my job" is not enough. "Meaningful" is defined by the team's recognition. In the traditional practice "meaningful" is defined by the doctor, never by the staff; in the new leadership style the participative process is defined by the team, with only the outcomes being critical to the leaders.

Sense of Involvement

Helping to do a job is not involvement; the team must be included in the decision process. Again, it is not something that happens *to them*—there are choices; victims cannot exist within a team. The width of the track is wide, and the milestones are clear, but it is the staff's accountability to get there—in time, with the required assets—that reflects involvement.

Feeling of Influence

Whereas the two previous components both enhance a feeling of influence in the individual, it is the team that influences the practice. Improvements and changes by team members are a continuous process; the staff have the ability to alter what is happening. If the team can create the environment, they will be able to cope with the stresses that occur in daily healthcare delivery.

Psychological Ownership

This is where the action is! The investment in the practice yields feelings of ownership; what is happening is theirs to control. The team accepts responsibility, with authority, and with accountability; the pride of this ownership is perceived by clients as *quality*.

Current literature on management places a great value on commitment, but it appears that no one has told those in the veterinary profession that commitment is a two-way street. The practice owner who has disposable staff will not get commitment. The owner who does not allow job sharing or variable schedules among staff members does not really want commitment to a purpose; that owner just wants someone to do the assigned job. A process-based control fanatic will not understand the description that follows.

The Highs and Lows

Countless workshops claim to teach managers how to create high commitment, how to build optimal performers, and how to make exceptional productivity occur within an average practice. In veterinary medicine, commitment is critical to retaining healthcare providers. This hype about commitment is not merely a management program; it is a product of leadership attention to purpose, job role, caring feedback mechanisms, and continuous collaborative improvement. Commitment and productivity are interrelated, but the extremes are bad news, as illustrated by Figure 2.2.

The graph uses 1 to 10 on the vertical productivity scale, and I show no one ever reaching a 10. This paradigm is a personal leadership philosophy based on continuous quality improvement; the world is changing too fast for anyone ever to be perfect. A true leader's job is to nurture others to achieve more within the parameters of their strengths and desires. In veterinary practice, productivity could be termed "the ability to bring clients back"; without that ability the practice cannot survive. Again, remember the basic premise of commitment: the team is there to facilitate the overall purpose of the practice, to do something that the team leader cannot do on his or her own. When the team becomes impaired because of an overzealous team member, the results can be poor information and poor sharing of insights.

The high-end commitment yields lower productivity because that is what we call burnout. At the high end of practice commitment lie the accidents: the too-fast pace, the divorces (almost half), and the high staff turnover rates. At high commitment, group think replaces individual innovation and creativity; personal observations and values are replaced by the required buy-in to the practice habits. The workaholic behavior makes the high-

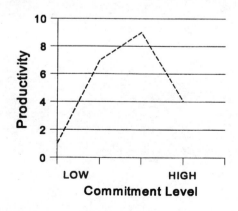

Fig. 2.2. Highs and lows of commitment

commitment person blind to team member needs and causes an inability to read the client or to assess the practice evolution from a critical viewpoint. Stasis sets in and compliance replaces improvement.

That is why the model shown at the beginning of this section is built on the concept of continuous collaborative improvement. Commitment is dependent upon the other components: purpose, alignment, feedback, and improvement are critical for maintaining high levels of commitment. Most traditional practice managers are not ready to listen, release control, or change. It is the uncommon leader who understands that you must let go of the present to grasp for the next rung on the ladder to success. Or, in the woods, you must release the tree trunk to go out on the limb.

Team TPR Evaluation Survey

Using the scale below, circle your response to the right of each item. The top-scale rates "what is"; the second scale rates "what is desired." This is an evaluation survey that requires maximum participation.

KEY: 1 - Not at all
2 - To a very little degree
3 - To a minor degree
4 - To a moderate degree
5 - To a significant degree
6 - To an outstanding degree

Purpose and Vision—*To what degree . . .*

1. are team members aware of the purpose, objectives, and goals?

   1 2 3 4 5 6 (Is)
   1 2 3 4 5 6 (Desired)

2. does this practice project a clear vision of its future?

   1 2 3 4 5 6 (Is)
   1 2 3 4 5 6 (Desired)

3. does this practice attempt to promote and explain a clear set of values?

   1 2 3 4 5 6 (Is)
   1 2 3 4 5 6 (Desired)

4. do personal values of the individual team members fit those of this practice?

   1 2 3 4 5 6 (Is)
   1 2 3 4 5 6 (Desired)

5. does the team mission support the overall mission of the practice?

   1 2 3 4 5 6 (Is)
   1 2 3 4 5 6 (Desired)

Roles—*To what degree . . .*

1. are team members knowledgeable about their roles and responsibilities?

   1 2 3 4 5 6 (Is)
   1 2 3 4 5 6 (Desired)

2. are team members in agreement with their roles and responsibilities?

   1 2 3 4 5 6 (Is)
   1 2 3 4 5 6 (Desired)

3. do team member roles contribute to the overall effectiveness of the practice?

   1 2 3 4 5 6 (Is)
   1 2 3 4 5 6 (Desired)

4. do the members of the team agree on standards of competent performance?　1 2 3 4 5 6 (Is)　1 2 3 4 5 6 (Desired)

5. are team members clear about how their roles/responsibilities relate to one another?　1 2 3 4 5 6 (Is)　1 2 3 4 5 6 (Desired)

6. are members of the team able to deal with ambiguity and changes?　1 2 3 4 5 6 (Is)　1 2 3 4 5 6 (Desired)

Feedback—*To what degree . . .*

1. does the team receive timely feedback on expected outcomes?　1 2 3 4 5 6 (Is)　1 2 3 4 5 6 (Desired)

2. do team members understand how they are contributing to the practice?　1 2 3 4 5 6 (Is)　1 2 3 4 5 6 (Desired)

3. is the team satisfied with the information received regarding its performance?　1 2 3 4 5 6 (Is)　1 2 3 4 5 6 (Desired)

4. do the members of the team get asked their opinions on a regular basis?　1 2 3 4 5 6 (Is)　1 2 3 4 5 6 (Desired)

5. are team member problems acknowledged and resolved?　1 2 3 4 5 6 (Is)　1 2 3 4 5 6 (Desired)

6. are practice challenges and problems acknowledged and resolved?　1 2 3 4 5 6 (Is)　1 2 3 4 5 6 (Desired)

7. is the team effort acknowledged and rewarded for accomplishments?　1 2 3 4 5 6 (Is)　1 2 3 4 5 6 (Desired)

Commitment—*To what degree . . .*

1. are team members willing to put forward the extra effort, beyond what is expected?　1 2 3 4 5 6 (Is)　1 2 3 4 5 6 (Desired)

2. do team members feel a strong loyalty to the practice?　1 2 3 4 5 6 (Is)　1 2 3 4 5 6 (Desired)

3. are team members inspired by the practice leadership to do their best?

1 2 3 4 5 6 (Is)
1 2 3 4 5 6 (Desired)

4. does the practice leadership outwardly invest in the team members?

1 2 3 4 5 6 (Is)
1 2 3 4 5 6 (Desired)

5. do team members have meaningful participation in the team?

1 2 3 4 5 6 (Is)
1 2 3 4 5 6 (Desired)

6. do team members have an ability to influence the direction of the practice?

1 2 3 4 5 6 (Is)
1 2 3 4 5 6 (Desired)

Collaboration—*To what degree . . .*

1. do members of the team display truth telling to one another?

1 2 3 4 5 6 (Is)
1 2 3 4 5 6 (Desired)

2. do team members trust communication and information received within the team?

1 2 3 4 5 6 (Is)
1 2 3 4 5 6 (Desired)

3. do team members blame one another or the practice for problems?

1 2 3 4 5 6 (Is)
1 2 3 4 5 6 (Desired)

4. do the members of the team have respect for one another?

1 2 3 4 5 6 (Is)
1 2 3 4 5 6 (Desired)

5. are team members encouraged to be innovative?

1 2 3 4 5 6 (Is)
1 2 3 4 5 6 (Desired)

6. does this practice look for ways to continually improve its effectiveness?

1 2 3 4 5 6 (Is)
1 2 3 4 5 6 (Desired)

7. is the team effort making a worthwhile contribution to the practice?

1 2 3 4 5 6 (Is)
1 2 3 4 5 6 (Desired)

THE FRAMEWORK FLOW

KNOWLEDGE—SKILLS—ATTITUDE

↓

EFFECTIVE LEADER

↓

STAFF- AND CLIENT-CENTERED
PROGRAMS, ACTION, POLICY

↓

QUALITY-BASED
HEALTHCARE DELIVERY

↓

SUPERVISION AND
OUTCOME ACCOUNTABILITY

↓

RECOGNITION AND CELEBRATION

↓

EFFECTIVE
VETERINARY PRACTICE

■ ■ ■ Review ■ ■ ■

In this chapter we have studied the definition of leadership, the traits of leadership, leadership principles (which include the 14 basic leadership skills). In addition, you have been given a self-evaluation of your own leadership qualities. Be sure you understand the material in this lesson before you proceed to Chapter 3: Closing in the Structure.

1. Veterinary Practice Leadership:
    The art of influencing and directing others in such a way as to obtain their willing participation, confidence, respect, and loyalty in order to serve the client, care for the patient, and enhance the practice.

2. Practice Leader Responsibilities:
    a. Accomplish the practice mission.
    b. Ensure the welfare of the staff.
    c. Establish a community market niche.

3. Leader's Actions:
    a. Accomplish one, two, or three of the leader's basic responsibilities.
    b. Be guided by the principles and skills of effective leadership.
    c. Take advantage of personal strengths and core values.

4. The 14 Skills of Leadership are based on personal qualities that nurture and esteem the individual and his or her team, thus gaining the willing participation, confidence, respect, and loyalty of team members in accomplishing the practice mission:
    a. Know and Use the Resources of the Group
    b. Effective Communication
    c. Understanding the Characteristics and Needs of the Group
    d. Reflection
    e. Representing the Group
    f. Effective Teaching
    g. Evaluating
    h. Planning
    i. Internal Promotion
    j. Situational Leadership
    k. Group Development
    l. Personal Relationships
    m. Setting the Example
    n. Continuous Quality Improvement

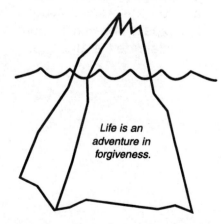

Life is an adventure in forgiveness.

5. Indications of Positive Practice Leadership:
   a. *Morale* is the state of mind of the individual. This personal perception is dependent upon the individual's attitude toward everything that affects him or her.
   b. *Harmony* is the individual or group attitude that ensures prompt co-operation and appropriate action in the absence of policy.
   c. *Esprit de corps* is the loyalty to, pride in, and enthusiasm for a practice shown by its members.
   d. *Proficiency* is the technical skill and knowledge, personal attitude, and physical ability of the individual and the practice team to achieve excellence.
   e. *An effective practice* is one in which, with the minimum expenditure of means and time, the team accomplishes any mission, assigned or implied, for which it has been organized, equipped, and trained.

6. Leadership Principles:
   a. Maintain technical and professional proficiency; train others to do the same.
   b. Know yourself and seek self-improvement regularly.
   c. Support your staff and look out for their welfare.
   d. Keep the team informed of the "why" and striving for improvement.
   e. Be consistent and set the example at all times.
   f. Ensure that the tasking is understood, supervised, and accomplished.
   g. Train individuals to a level of trust as well as task-based competence.
   h. Make sound and timely decisions in healthcare and in staff leadership.
   i. Develop a sense of responsibility within the team and recognize their efforts.
   j. Assign projects based on capabilities of the individual.
   k. Personally seek responsibility and accept accountability.
   l. Expect excellence, pursue continuous quality improvement, and celebrate the attempts.

CHAPTER THREE

Closing in the Structure

The Glue to Hold It Together

The objective of leadership is to accomplish the mission in the minimum time and with the maximum balance of individual needs.
— *Dr. T. E. Cat*

Styles of Leadership

Too often leaders focus their efforts on short-range goals at the unnecessary expense of their subordinates (the team is subordinate to the leader but does not need to be made to feel that way). In the long run this can be detrimental to both the staff and the practice. Effective leadership means accomplishing the mission with a minimum expenditure of personal time and effort and an appropriate balance between practice, staff, and individual needs and goals.

Leadership ability becomes increasingly important as the practice team expands. When the practice becomes a multipractitioner healthcare delivery system, leadership becomes a prerequisite for team building and success. Although there are many styles of leadership, with shades of gray in the spectrum of good approaches, nearly all can be classed as either directive or nondirective leadership methods.

• The directive leader tells the staff exactly what to do and lets them know who is the boss. Group members have the security of knowing exactly what is expected of them. This is critical when a new task or new member is added to the team; it is called training.

• Nondirective leaders seek the opinions of team members, consult with them in planning and decision making, and sometimes, on nonhealthcare issues, even put ideas to a democratic vote. Although this isn't the best idea in case management, in practice management it is essential for growth.

• Team members may vary by practice and by the moment. Situations of stress, whether they be patient needs or client demands, cause interactions among team members to vary. A leader must be tuned in to the tone of the moment to understand which style of leadership is needed in a given situation.

• In diagrammatic explanation, the styles of leadership can be shown on a sliding scale, with positive staff development on one axis, and the leader's behavior on the other (See Figure 3.1).

Match the Context

No one approach (leadership style) is appropriate at all times. In general, directive styles will be more appropriate in life-saving situations and when training starter-level employees. The new team member deserves to know what is expected without having to guess or ask for a consensus; knowledge is power, and some don't share it well (especially the insecure staff member). The more participative style is for the mature team; it is used in team-building practice-management situations, and with competent professional and paraprofessional associates.

In short, Group Development can also be put on a two-axis diagram, with a double variable: new staff member feelings and new task knowledge on one axis, and time on the other axis (see Figure 3.2). We assume

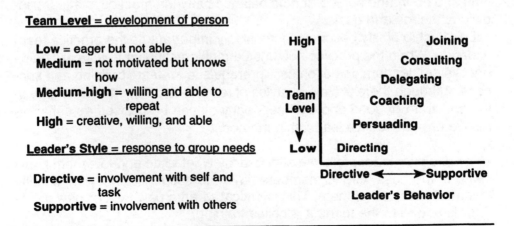

Fig. 3.1. Styles of leadership

* = relationships (morale)

0 = task effectiveness

Stage 1 = high relationships, low task effectiveness

Stage 2 = lowest relationships while effectiveness begins to increase

Stage 3 = relationships improving, task effectiveness getting better

Stage 4 = high relationships and highest task effectiveness

Forming	Storming	Norming	Performing
Stage 1	Stage 2	Stage 3	Stage 4

Fig. 3.2. Group development

that all new team members start with high morale (they are happy to be hired) and low practice-specific task knowledge (new people don't know where they fit into the practice pecking order, or how the practice operates on a daily basis):

There are four stages in most group development situations. Each of the stages can be understood from a logical and progressive standpoint, simply by looking at how the practice has usually approached tasks and how group needs were met. In fact, Stage 1 and Stage 2 can be shortened by an astute leader using the situational leadership styles, but they cannot be eliminated. Harmony comes with shortening the Stage 1 and Stage 2 phases, so please consider the following:

Stage 1—Forming

Task - The team usually can't do it, so they spend effort on defining goals, planning the approach, and evaluating the resources not currently available.

Group - The team is dependent upon the leader and anxious about who they are, why they are there, what they'll get, where they fit in relation to the leader's role, if they'll be liked, and what the group goals mean to them. They have positive expectations and

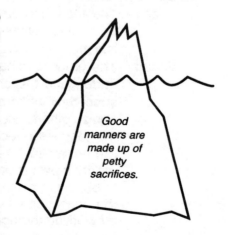

Good manners are made up of petty sacrifices.

moderate eagerness. (This stage is task and teaching dependent: how clear is the task, how well prepared are the staff, and
how easy does it seem?)

Stage 2—Storming

Task - Team skills are improving, so some accomplishment occurs,
some negative feelings about must-do tasks and following the
leader.

Group - Reality is different from the team's original hopes and expectations, the differences are unsatisfying, and nerves are tense.
Some are dissatisfied with their position in the pecking order or
with the leader. They question ever wanting the job; they react
negatively with anger, frustration, and feelings of incompe-
tence or confusion. (A caring leader needs to shorten this
phase by redefining projects into very small can-do tasks.)

Stage 3—Norming

Task - The group can do it, but slowly, while building their confidence.
They have a positive approach to problem solving, and the
ability to complete projects.

Group - The team discovers how to work together to make tasks easier and fun. Personal differences are resolving, accomplishment brings pride; there is less animosity, more mutual respect, better trust, greater unity, growing self-esteem, and a
feeling of belonging. (This is a short stage in professional
groups, but a long stage for most staff groups unless dissatis-
factions are resolved, new skills are learned, bonding occurs,
and recognition of good work is frequent.)

Stage 4—Performing

Task - The team can perform the task easily, with efficiency, knowledge, and confidence. There is pride in the outcome and satisfaction in the process.

Group - The group is cohesive, unified, eager to be a team. Members
understand the characteristics and needs of each other, respect their differences, challenge and support each other, recognize others' accomplishments, feel capable of acting without
the leader's direction, have open and free communications,
are not afraid of rejection, feel confident about outcomes, create their own tasks, fill in each other's weaknesses, and want
to belong to a can-do team. (This stage will last until the end of
the project or activity, or until staff are realigned; it comes only
by working through other stages.)

There Is a Stage 5—It Is Called Termination.
This occurs when the task or group comes to an end. Group effectiveness either falls apart or increases to meet deadlines and demands. Group members feel a sense of loss, a sadness about the separation, and a concern about the future. They hide their feelings with jokes or expressions of dissatisfaction (frustration) but have a pride and strong positive feeling about the past. (This is the team-rebuilding phase all leaders must face.)

Remember the styles of leadership (Figure 3.1)? Please compare these two figures; lay them atop each other. Note how the more directive styles are used to shorten Stage 1 (directing and persuading) and Stage 2 (persuading and coaching). Try to describe, in your own terms, which styles become important in each of the stages in your own practice experience.

Take a special look at the uses of the different styles of leadership:

Stage 1 - directing ➜ persuading (Get them to buy into ownership of outcomes.)

Stage 2 - persuading ➜ coaching (Build confidence in personal abilities.)

Stage 3 - coaching ➜ delegating and consulting (Reinforce good work, proficiency, skills, and competency.)

Stage 4 - consulting ➜ joining (This is fun time—working within the group for better results.)

Summarizing research, models, and theories developed by a variety of social scientists, Professor Chemers of Claremont McKenna College gives this advice: "If your subordinates do not have the knowledge necessary to perform the task, or if their attitude is such that they lack commitment to the goal at hand, a directive approach is warranted." The most common example of this situation is a chemotherapeutic regimen for a patient wherein the drug, dose, duration, and administration are dictated by the veterinarian.

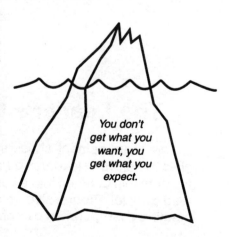

You don't get what you want, you get what you expect.

Of course, even the best veterinarian doesn't always have a clear picture of what the most desirable course of treatment should be. You may need a colleague's perspective or the staff's ability to provide subjective information on the case or client; here participation is called for. When a veterinarian is nondirective, it is more likely that the team members' intellectual abilities, years of practical experience, or technical capabilities will contribute to the task. This is especially true for challenges in practice management that deal with client bonding or improving productivity.

The participative style has some important bonuses. It makes team members feel autonomous—a proved motivator for some personality types—and it gives them the opportunity to develop their skills. In deciding between the two schools of leadership, also consider the bottom line—Can subordinates be expected to energetically implement a management decision if they didn't participate in making it? Developing the reward system for profit-based performance standards is an example of this concept in action.

Many veterinary practices automatically assume that pay raises, bonuses, and other monetary rewards are the only way to increase job satisfaction and productivity. With the salary budget getting tighter every year, you've got to find other ways to motivate and reward your staff members.

In veterinary healthcare many individual staff members want recognition for their achievements. (You can be sure they are not in our profession for the money.) This recognition can take the form of new, more challenging assignments, greater job visibility, and the opportunity to interact with clients and patients. Don't make the mistake of treating all your staff members the same. Design a reward and recognition system that truly meets each staff member's needs.

> *The obscure we eventually see ... the completely obvious,*
> *it seems, takes longer.*
> — *Edward R. Murrow*

The Leader's Management Checklist

This management checklist is actually a leadership checklist that applies the skills of leadership (*Managing from the Heart*, by Hyler Bracey, et al., puts this concept into a caring perspective). We *manage* programs; we *lead* people. Progressive veterinary practices have leaders causing and creating change (often perceived as chaos by traditionalists) on a daily basis; they empower their team members to contribute ideas. They take the restrictions off the backs of people who want to use innovation and creativity to better meet client and practice needs, and they put traditional controls on those who blame or want to maintain the status quo; the latter type of staff member kills a practice in today's environment. Here are nine leadership skill applications, most of which will fit most practices:

Start with Core Values and a Single Standard

The practice leader must be predictable. The *core values* are six or so tenets that will never be violated—principles that others can make decisions upon and never catch heat from the boss. The *single standard* means that anyone who excels for the good of the practice, or anyone who violates a hospital value or policy, will be treated equally, good or bad—no favorites when handing out recognitions, punishments, or rewards.

Level with Individuals

If there is not adequate cash flow in the practice to give monetary rewards, say so. Advise staff members what they must do to survive; be candid. They will discover the truth soon enough.

Be Vocal About Strong Points

Stress the positive benefits of success. Hold back discussing shortcomings unless they are doing damage to the practice. If a discussion concerning certain areas that need improvement is likely to improve matters, do it in private when things are calm and quiet.

Express Appreciation for Small Tasks Well Done

Evaluate the success of each new plan or effort. Keep an eye on the progress made by the individual. You can afford to ignore small tasks that are done poorly, but you need to act in a timely manner for appreciation and recognition to be meaningful. Advertise a person's good performance.

Offer Your Personal Assistance

If you think a staff member will be helped by adding your effort, do so if he or she is willing to accept your aid. Offer the vital resources needed, without strings attached, to get the job done properly. This could mean anything from supplying muscle, food, telephone time, or other forms of assistance.

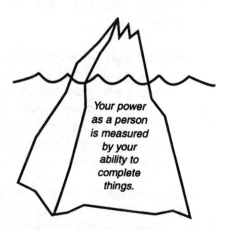

Your power as a person is measured by your ability to complete things.

Listen to Dissenters

Try to do something *for,* not *about,* the individual. Involve yourself with people, not cliques.

Let Team Members Make Decisions

Be liberal with information about the desired outcomes and the resource limitations or parameters of the program; this will help the staff do a better job or come up with alternatives for improving their personal areas of work interest.

Promise Only What Is Certain

If you *think* you can deliver, be quiet. If you are *sure* you can deliver, use that promise to build excitement and the dream.

Make People Feel Like Winners

✔ Reward solid solutions to ensure the achievement of long-range goals and objectives.

✔ Reward risk taking, applied creativity, and decisive action to boost the feeling of belonging.

✔ Reward smart work, simplification, quietly effective behavior, and quality work to improve productivity.

✔ Reward loyalty and working together to foster teamwork and cooperation.

Designing Recognitions and Rewards

Here are another nine applications of the common leadership skills that should be considered when developing recognitions and rewards. If you want a great paperback text for your library, the book by Michael LeBoeuf, *The Greatest Management Principle in the World—GMP,* expands on the following ideas:

Distinguish Between High Performers and Low Producers

Movement is not always progress. Trying to increase overall performance with a system that rewards everyone equally for compliance with a set of guidelines does nothing to motivate high producers or to sustain their exceptional level of performance or ability to solve problems independently. Recognition is one of the top three reasons staff members join a veterinary practice; be targeted and specific.

Distinguish Between Rewards That Retain People and Those That Encourage Higher Productivity

There is a difference, such as the traditional merit pay system based on tenure and inflation, as opposed to one based on superior performance. A technician who demonstrates the ability to perform as a paraprofessional veterinary extender, capable of providing enhanced service to clients, is a prime candidate for recognition based on outstanding performance. Your respect should be followed immediately by overt recognition for exceeding expectations; thus individual responsibility is assigned as a very special form of reward.

Ask Employees What Kinds of Rewards They Would Like and Be Specific About What You Can Offer

Someone who is achievement oriented might want more challenging work. An affiliation-oriented person might desire being put in charge of an inventory management team. A power-oriented individual might desire greater visibility, such as a new title posted on a letter board in the reception area. By finding out what motivates each employee and setting up a more personal reward system, you can enhance job satisfaction as well as personal performance.

Put Reward Opportunities in Writing

Staff members will be more likely to respond when they are assured that a known standard for a reward or recognition is measurable, will be delivered as promised, and is beyond the routine expectations of the practice. Some practices even have a contest of the month, just to bring attention to healthcare delivery areas or client/patient programs needing emphasis.

Reserve Some Rewards for the Team

When building a team composed of professionals and paraprofessionals, the problem of dual standards will always arise. The astute leader will develop a recognition system (thank-you method) that acknowledges team effort, as well as individual systems to recognize high performers. Do not forget: families (and significant others) support the practice also; a quarterly social event is appropriate just to say thanks to them. Not all teams have a lineup of stars, but even the best quarterback requires a solid and dependable line to score!

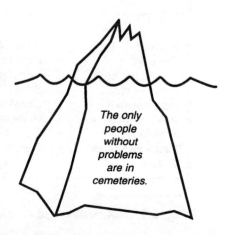

The only people without problems are in cemeteries.

Don't Offer Rewards That Are Meaningful Only to the Practice

When a work enthusiast takes on an extremely challenging job single-handedly, he or she experiences an adrenaline rush. That doesn't mean all the staff members want to go out on a limb alone, nor does it mean they have the same motivation. Make sure you don't get blinded by your own assessment of practice needs when deciding what kind of things will motivate your staff.

When Giving Verbal Praise, Make It Timely, Specific, and Sincere

Do not try walking up to a staff member three weeks after the fact and merely saying that he or she did well. Catch a person right after a project, specify what you liked, then link adjectives like "creative," "caring," and "bright" to your recognition.

Don't Dilute Praise with Qualifications

When praising and recognizing members of the team, leave the words "but," "otherwise," and "if" out of the discussion. Also, do not use recognition as a punishment for others who did not excel; this will inevitably result in the recipient's enduring retaliatory behavior from the peer group. Praise the intent of the action, not the results.

Don't Reward the Wrong Behavior

The 11 most common ways to *recognize appropriate behavior* are outlined in Figure 3.3.

How to Use Cash Rewards

The most commonly seen problem is the practice owner/manager learning how to define the desired end results … and creating the environment

Use This Reward	To Reward This Behavior	Instead of This Behavior
*Recognition	Risk Taking	Risk Avoiding
*Fun	Loyalty	Turnover
*Money	Solid Solutions	Quick Fixes
*Time Off	Applied Creativity	Mindless Conformity
*Profit Sharing	Decisive Action	Paralysis of Analysis
*Favorite Work	Smart Work	Busy Work
*Advancement	Simplification	Needless Complications
*Position Title	Problem Solution	Problem Identification
*Freedom	Quiet Effectiveness	Squeaky Wheel
*Personal Growth	Quality Work	Fast Work
*Prizes	Working Together	Working Against Each Other

Fig. 3.3. Rewarding appropriate behavior

required for others to achieve them. The term "cash incentive" or "cash bonus" is a misnomer in veterinary medicine; we do not pay enough initially to believe the team members aren't "earning" every penny they get! Please call the earned extra monies "management fees," "productivity pay," "performance pay," or even "recognition pay." The following are a few alternatives to start considering:

Inventory Management Fee. Two technicians form an inventory management team with a recognition management fee of 20 percent of the savings under the projected cash budget as computed quarterly. A typical scenario is a 15 percent cost of drugs and medical supplies (without laboratory, imaging, or nutritional goods) with a 13 percent target by end of year, which requires a 0.5 percent decrease in expenditure each quarter. For our illustration, a 13 percent cost in drugs and medical supplies would earn the team a 20 percent share of the 2 percent savings in the total drug and medical supply expense during the first quarter, a 1.5 percent share the second quarter, and decreasing savings the third or fourth quarter. In reality, the lower return in the second quarter would alert the team to the trend and would likely cause additional corrective action on their part before the third quarter.

Appointment Log Fill Rate. Days when the log has greater than an 80 percent exam room fill, based on available facilities (exam rooms, not doctors), the receiving team gets 20 percent of the extra fill rate income (computed daily) in a monthly recognition bonus, as illustrated by a 90 percent fill on a $2,000 income day: 90 percent − 80 percent = 10 percent; therefore 10 percent × $2,000 = $200, then 20 percent of $200 = the receiving team's portion of about $40.

Staff Productivity Recognition. According to the annual cash budget, a percentage of gross is committed for staff salaries (nondoctor), to be measured quarterly. In quarters during which there has been short staffing, or excess practice growth, the staff percentage computation and comparison will show an actual cash savings; this savings is divided among the staff. A suggested division is 10 percent for the scheduling team, 40 percent for the staff (shares equitably determined by the scheduling team), and 30 percent for the staff Christmas stocking (end-of-year bonus); this leaves the practice about 20 percent for tax requirement purposes.

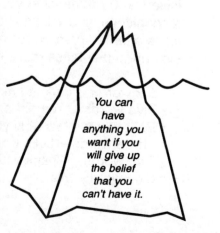

You can have anything you want if you will give up the belief that you can't have it.

Practice Manager Performance Management Fee. The difference between income and expense on the P&L (Profit & Loss Statement, also called Income Statement) is called "net." The term "excess net" is based on the cash budget projections (which include rent, ROI [Return on Investment], reasonable clinical salaries for all doctors, and balance sheet monies) on a quarterly basis. Excess net (on the P&L) can be caused by either (1) producing extra income (e.g., paraprofessional outreach programs, recalls, promotions) or (2) increasing cost control (e.g., reduced overtime, better control of stockage levels, economies of scale purchases with other practices). When the staff and programs are managed by a staff person, the practice manager can be recognized with 20 percent of the excess net as a management fee, illustrated as follows:

If $6,000 quarterly net is the target and $10,000 is the actual net for the quarter, the quarterly excess net is $4,000. The manager's recognition management fee (20 percent) would be $800 (while the practice retains $3,200 of the unexpected excess net).

The Importance of Effective Communication

Regardless of leadership styles or recognition/reward systems, the secret is to communicate effectively. This means that information is given and received in each exchange. Brains and ambition are hard to recognize and reward if they are muffled by lackluster or annoying verbal traits. It does not matter how brilliant or sincere an individual is; if the message doesn't come across verbally, it will be lost.

When your staff believe that you have confidence in them, they will be more likely to present new ideas, do higher-quality work, and take more initiative. By reinforcing your belief in the practice staff with rewards and recognitions, you will find yourself managing an aggressive rather than a crisis-oriented practice team. To keep your profit-based efforts in perspective, try to use these most important words frequently:

- Six words - "I admit I made a mistake."
- Five words - "You did a good job."
- Four words - "What is your opinion?"
- Three words - "Let's work together."
- Two words - "Thank you."
- One word - "We."

Filters of Communication

Information is processed at various levels of understanding. Based on the mind-set of the listener, it flows through the experiences of the past and is thus distorted. Every person has these filters, so additions and deletions are made based on the listener's interpretation. Some of the more common filters encountered in practice leadership situations include:

- What the leader *believes* he or she heard, either verbally or in writing. Clarification of the communicator's intent is rarely sought.

- What the leader believes the staff should know, for their own good or for protection of the practice.

- What the leader believes the staff wants to hear, regardless of the practice needs or environmental situation.

- What the leader thinks should be toned down or built up for the benefit of the receiver. Facts are mutable.

- What the leader's values and attitudes do to the information—the bias of prejudice and personal ethics.

- What stress or stresses the leader is operating under, at home or in the practice.

- What importance the leader attaches to the information, ignoring the validity of perceptions other than his or her own.

- What the leader is feeling at the moment the information is being received or when passing the information to others.

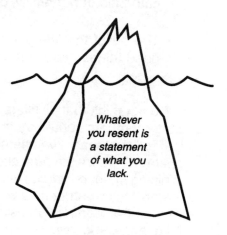

Whatever you resent is a statement of what you lack.

When we consider the filters that information must pass through at each level, it is understandable that distortion, dilution, or total loss of understanding occurs. Do not, indeed, misunderstand these comments—after all, it is the leader's *job* to filter messages in order to clarify them or add to them as required. The leader, however, should not allow personal feelings and stresses to filter communications inappropriately or covertly.

The downward flow of information has the practice's seal of approval behind it. A kind of gravity flow exists. On the other hand, feedback is critical to ensure that communication has occurred. Remember, both the giving *and* the getting of information is essential for effective team communications. The average veterinary healthcare delivery team also filters information in the communication process. Many of the staff filters are even more severe and cutting than those applied to downward communication, making meaningful feedback even more difficult. Some common filters that staff members apply to upward communications are:

- The notion that any opinion in opposition to the boss's idea is negative thinking and therefore bad.

- The notion that practice teams always gripe, and the manager will worry only when they don't.

- The belief that the manager will assume staff don't have the big picture in mind, and the feedback with, therefore, be unimportant.

- The belief that the veterinarian is not interested in the paraprofessional perception.

- The belief that a person will get into trouble for passing along certain information.

- The belief that the information will reflect adversely on the communicator, his or her ability, or the staff effort.

- The belief that the practice manager/owner wants to be told only the good things and not the bad things.

Do not think that all filters are bad. Some filters serve a useful purpose. Staff members should try to solve problems or, when addressing a problem, offer at least two alternative solutions. They need to take the appropriate action, try the best alternatives, and pass on significant information. Whining is not constructive communication. The acid test for staff is to ask themselves whether they would need or like to have the information if they were in the leadership position. They should pass the information on only if the answer is yes.

Bridges to Communication

Some guidelines for communicating more effectively using either style of leadership are:

- Keep it short, simple, and direct.

- Word your questions so that they will elicit a "yes" response. Your position is then associated with the positive.

- Suit your message to the audience.

- Use words like "let's" to associate yourself automatically with the team.

- Use a story or anecdote as a window. Construct a vivid scenario of "what if" or "when" to make the team imagine the events already occurring.

- Using words like "right" or "truth" puts your position on the positive side of a debate.

- Know when not to speak. A dramatic pause after a particularly important point will stress your sincerity. It also allows you to evaluate how your message is being received. If you are negotiating, present your case, then leave in silence.

Improving your own communication skills to meet the needs required to cope with varying leadership styles is only smart business. Select those things you can affect, and do your best to be all you can be with those things you can influence. Do not spend great amounts of time fretting over things you cannot influence; focusing on the doable makes for a far better practice environment. Through an awareness of the filters and barriers in the practice's communication systems, a leader can decide which communication system can be used, how to reduce the effects of the filters, and where to look should breakdowns occur. Good communication does not just happen—it must be developed and maintained by each and every team leader.

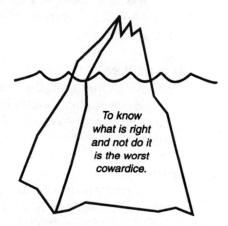

To know
what is right
and not do it
is the worst
cowardice.

An important facet of any leader's responsibility for developing and maintaining effective communications is that of daily coaching and counseling. The veterinary healthcare team wants to be better. They want to give the best to the clients and patients. Communication is the most significant means of influencing team members' behavior, their self-image and self-worth, and their participation in the practice's goals and objectives. Remember, we are each 100 percent responsible for sending a clear message to others so they can understand what we're trying to communicate.

Planning Should Mean Putting It Together Right

The ability to use the 14 leadership skills and the multiple principles shared in Chapter 2 means that *advanced* planning will occur in a systematic method. In veterinary practice we must be ready to react to the emergency, but a good planning process reduces this necessity outside the healthcare delivery arena. The challenge is usually where to start (or, in some cases, making the time to start, but that is another issue). Let's add structure to this process:

Task
Determine the activity, set the objective, clearly define the issues.
What is the purpose? Why do it? What is gained?
What—When—Where—Why—Who—How! ! !

Resources
What are the available resources to the practice team?
Are the resources readily available? Are there restrictions in their use?
Time—Skills—Equipment—People—Community—Money—References! ! !

Alternatives
Based on the available resources, what alternatives are available?
There are multiple ways to accomplish every task; brainstorm them.
Emergencies?—Weather?—Economy?—Fun?—Pride?—Client Access?

Specifics
The activity must be planned for the details, so write it down in detail.
Every Plan A must have a Plan B as backup.
Date?—Time?—Place?—Assignments?—Success Measurements?

Implementation

Initiate the plan; stay centered on desired outcomes, not process.
Follow the plan, but be ready to make changes in the process to get to the outcome.
Just do it!

Evaluation

How did the activity go? Were objectives met? How was success measured?
Should we do it again? What could we improve?
Recognition of special efforts—reward appropriate behavior and effort.

• THE LAST STEP is actually the first step of the new planning process!

Review the six steps in Figure 3.4. and assess which of the 14 leadership skills are involved in the planning process. An astute evaluation will show that all the leadership skills are involved, at different levels of intensity, depending on the plan developed by the team. Where did the veterinarian's oath fit into the planning process? Was the oath a characteristic, a need, a resource, a reflection, or did it just form the core values of the thought process? Does the veterinarian's oath meet the definition of "discovery," or was it part of the teaching/learning evaluation? How does it help develop the group in your practice, and how does it influence your styles of leadership in the personal relationships of the practice? What example are you setting as you continually strive to improve?

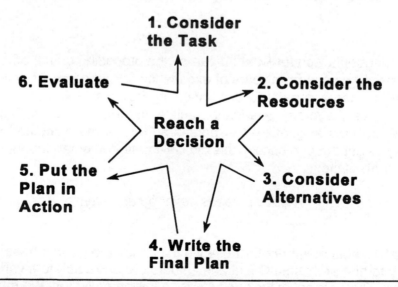

Fig. 3.4. Remember the five P's: prior planning prevents poor performance

The first question most practice team members will ask is "Who is responsible?" The answer is always, "The leader is responsible." Making no decision is, in fact, a decision, and that is a leader's choice. A poor decision is better than no decision if the leader allows other people the freedom to change the process to meet the desired outcomes. Group decisions lead to buy-in, although in cases of health, safety, and money allocation, the leader must react (situational leadership) without the team's consensus. Leadership means sharing the "why" in the initial phases of planning, along with the What—When—Where—Who—and—How.

Planning is essential to getting the job done while holding the group together. Veterinary practice happens as it should if the team plans carefully and then gets to carry out the plans. Participation is based on commitments during the planning process; verbal rehearsals allow the staff to interact and refine the ideas *before* writing them down. Do you ever use the oral rehearsal? Like talking to the mirror? This skill is also critical for doctors when looking at optimum care for patients. Rehearse client narratives without using the words "recommend," "better than," "should consider," which make healthcare optional. Use "animals deserve" or "patient needs" or even "I need." (When was the last time your staff ceased to participate in a new program because there was no active involvement in the planning process?)

A New Method for Staff Evaluation

The veterinarian earns the gross, but the staff makes the net.
—Dr. T. E. Cat

Some people wonder what I mean by the preceding quote; others take it as insight gained from years of experience in management. It is only a commonsense approach to understanding how valuable the healthcare delivery team is to any veterinary practice. In Montana, where Bob Miller taught me how to gentle-break horses and gave me a method to earn money to get through school, this old California horseman taught me one basic truth of life:

"A good horse is never a bad color."

We hire staff members because we think they are good horses. We do not try to hire problems. Our staff members are dedicated to a caring profession. They are not in the business for a million-dollar job. We must treat our staff like diamonds if we want our clients treated like diamonds. With a quality diamond, we change the setting to exhibit its best facets. We do not even think about changing the diamond.

The veterinarian can generate gross income by laying hands upon animals, but it is a receptionist who converts a phone call into a client, a technician who recalls a client and converts him or her into a return visit, and an animal caretaker who bathes an animal so well that the client tells her neighbors of the great service of the hospital. The staff makes most of the client contacts, projecting everything from the facility image (inside and outside) to the tone of communications. As Karyn Gavzer pointed out in the October 1991 cover article of the *AVMA Marketing and Practice Strategies*, increasing visit frequency is the most painless and profitable method to increase practice liquidity.

Evaluate the Staff Effort

Because the concept of staff evaluation usually brings terror to a practice manager's heart, we will provide alternatives. What I want each reader to do is evaluate the impact of his or her staff on the operations of the practice—measure the *right* things, as opposed to the average client transaction (ACT), which means virtually *nothing*. This can be done in at least four ways:

1. Calculate client visits per year.
2. Make fiscal comparisons.
3. Determine payroll costs.
4. Study turnover rates.

Calculate client visits per year —Most practices plan on multiple visits per year per client but do not track this trend as a management tool. New clients are often tracked, but new clients by existing client referral are not. Visits per pet per year are harder to retrieve than visits per client (except on a few computer systems), so they are seldom tracked. Each of these factors tells something about the client communication and bonding that occurs at any specific practice.

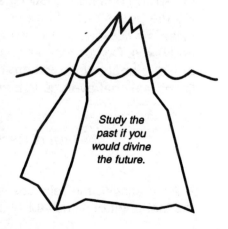

Study the past if you would divine the future.

Make fiscal comparisons—Some practices track the sales per full-time-equivalent veterinarian; fewer know the sales per full-time equivalent parapro-fessional. Table 3.1 (page 86) is a self-assessment worksheet to assist in comparing the payroll hours per transaction, a valuable productivity and performance management tool. It is an easy form to complete from already existing information, yet it evaluates the annual paraprofes-sional staff effort from a different perspective.

Determine payroll costs—In most studies of the value a practice places on supporting its staff, the benefits are often quoted but seldom shown by computation. The value of the benefits often needs to be put into per-spective for the staff to evaluate, especially during salary negotiations, so Table 3.2 (page 87) has been provided to reflect total payroll costs. In the U.S. government, this type of value exercise is done annually for every employee and provided to them individually at the beginning of the fiscal or calendar year. In some practices this is also done for vet-erinarians, and the veterinarian is allowed to adjust the benefit package figures internally, but still within the budget restriction of 20 to 23 percent of his or her personal production.

Study turnover rates—The cost of turnover rates is seldom computed, but the untrained receptionist does not effectively close the appointment sale or respond to the client's concern. These are costs that are never captured. The local chamber of commerce will generally provide you ex-pected turnover rates within certain segments of the community's pop-ulation, as will the state wage and labor authority. The turnover rate of a practice must be evaluated to assess the quality of service as well as the training costs. Table 3.3 will assist in this evaluation effort.

The trends in a specific practice are often missed because we look at the wrong numbers. Fiscal graphs help us assess the trends by compar-ing the peaks and valleys as well as the slopes on a common horizontal axis. The figures used for wages paid should include the benefit packages and taxes. Do not concern yourself with *national averages*. Instead, be im-pressed about what you are doing in your own practice. To keep a pub-lished national average in perspective, try to remember that it represents only

"the best of the worst or the worst of the best."

As practical, the relationship trends should be assessed starting from the last point of staff stability (in some practices this is a misnomer, as the management believes in a disposable staff). There are other charts that are possible to use, but the key data have been organized into the following tables for quick reference.

The Dirty Dozen Questions

When the worksheets are completed, an evaluation of the practice trends will be required. If the payroll is an increasing percentage of the gross income, then the gross income as well as the personnel costs must be evaluated prior to layoff action. In most cases, programs will require restructuring to increase the liquidity. If the payroll hours per transaction increase, then the number of transactions as well as staffing schedules must be evaluated before cutting the payroll hours. The dozen questions that need to be considered are in Table 3.4.

Table 3.1. Key Fiscal Comparisons

Key Factor	19__	19__	19__	19__
Total Income	_____	_____	_____	_____
Total # Transactions	_____	_____	_____	_____
Total Clients Seen	_____	_____	_____	_____
Average Transaction	_____	_____	_____	_____
Total Payroll	_____	_____	_____	_____
Percent Payroll of Income	_____	_____	_____	_____
Total Payroll Hours	_____	_____	_____	_____
Payroll Hours per Transaction	_____	_____	_____	_____

OTHER COMPARISONS POSSIBLE

Average Sales per FTE* Staff Member	_____	_____	_____	_____
Average Sales per FTE* Veterinarian	_____	_____	_____	_____

*Full-time-equivalent

Table 3.2. Total Payroll Costs

Annual Dollars Spent for:

Wages (time, overtime, premium pay, etc.)	$_____
Salaries (time, percentages, etc.)	$_____
Continuing Education Expenses	$_____
Workers' Compensation Insurance Premium (less rebate)	$_____
Social Security Payment (employer's share only)	$_____
Unemployment Compensation Payments	$_____
Group Insurance (net employer payments only)	$_____
Bonus Payments Not in Wage/Salary	$_____
Profit Sharing Payments (if any)	$_____
Pension Program (net employer payments only)	$_____
Vacation Pay (if not included in wage/salary)	$_____
Holiday Pay (if not included in wage/salary)	$_____
Uniform Expenses (with laundry as applicable)	$_____
Meal Subsidies (other than C.E.)	$_____
Cost of Locker Room/Employer Area (if exclusive use)	$_____
Other Personnel Costs (direct)	$_____
Total Employment Cost	$_____

Table 3.3. Turnover Rates

1. Who were the full-time-equivalent (FTE) staff?

	12 Months Ago	Today
Veterinarians	_____	_____
Receptionists	_____	_____
Technicians	_____	_____
Animal Caretakers	_____	_____
Groomers	_____	_____
Others	_____	_____

2. What was the rate of turnover during the last 12 months?

Moved away	_____
Got a "better" job	_____
Changed careers	_____
Discharged	_____
Quit	_____
Retired	_____
Married	_____
Other	_____
TOTAL	_____

3. Putting numbers to the assessment:

a = number of employees represented by each financial statement in the 12-month period

b = number of new employee positions added (and filled) to staff in that specific month for each month

c = average number of employees for year

$$c = \frac{a - b \text{ for each of the 12 months, then total all 12}}{12}$$

4. Turnover as percentage of our average number of employees:

$$\frac{\text{total of number 2 above x 100}}{\text{average number of employees (3c above)}}$$

5. What is the expected community turnover rate? _____

6. What is our desired turnover rate? _____

Table 3.4. The Dirty Dozen

If payroll is an increasing percentage of the gross income, or if the payroll hours per transaction are increasing, ask these questions:

1. Have our quarterly fee schedules kept current with the inflation rate and increases in other costs?

2. Did we increase our fees to support wage and salary increases?

3. Did any change in scope of services or technology cause the staffing increases/decreases, changes in individual or practice productivity, or higher/lower labor costs?

4. Was there a change in the turnover rate? Why did it occur? Did the exit interviews with departing staff support our assumptions on internal personnel relations?

5. Have we had a problem hiring quality personnel? Have we researched the real reasons for hiring less than top-quality staff?

6. Are there bad feelings between some staff members? Do some staff members seem uninterested in their work? Does this interfere with healthcare delivery or team harmony?

7. Are more staff members asking for raises? Are their wages/salaries competitive within the community (veterinary and nonveterinary)?

8. Are longer lunches, absenteeism, or tardiness increasing? Are staff members leaving work earlier?

9. Are staff members abusing break periods, vacation time, or sick days?

10. Do staff members have increasing behavior problems? Has more time been required to "keep people in line"?

11. What has the client's exit interview reflected? Are we losing clients because of dissatisfaction? Do their responses match our assumptions?

12. Have we used joint goal setting with individual staff members on a quarterly basis? Have goals been routinely met?

■ ■ ■ Review ■ ■ ■

In this lesson we've pointed out the difference between directive and nondirective leadership styles and when they are best used. We've also addressed how we all filter our communications with each other, and how to bridge communication gaps. You should now be able to determine your own leadership style and monitor your own communication filters. You may now proceed to Chapter 4: Inside Finishing.

1. Styles of Leadership:
   a. Stage 1—Directing to persuading (staff buying into ownership outcomes)
   b. Stage 2—Persuading to coaching (building staff confidence in abilities)
   c. Stage 3—Coaching to delegating and consulting recognizing staff proficiency, skills, and competency)
   d. Stage 4—Consulting to joining (working within the group for better results)

2. Stages of Group Development:
   a. Forming
   b. Storming
   c. Norming
   d. Performing
   e. Termination (optional)

3. Manager's Checklist:
   a. Start with core values and a single standard.
   b. Level with individuals.
   c. Be vocal about strong points.
   d. Express appreciation for small tasks well done.
   e. Offer your personal assistance.
   f. Listen to dissenters.
   g. Let team members make decisions.
   h. Promise only what is certain.
   i. Make people feel like winners.

4. Recognize the Appropriate Behaviors:
   a. Distinguish between high performers and low producers.
   b. Distinguish between rewards that retain people and those that will encourage higher productivity.

    c. Ask employees what kinds of rewards they would like and what you can offer.

    d. Put reward opportunities into writing.

    e. Reserve some rewards for the team.

    f. Don't offer rewards that are meaningful only within the practice.

    g. When giving verbal praise, make it timely, specific, and sincere.

    h. Do not dilute praise with qualifications.

    i. Don't reward the wrong behavior.

5. Bridges to Communication:
   a. Keep it short, simple, direct.
   b. Ask questions that elicit a "yes" response.
   c. Match message to audience.
   d. Use team-associated type words, like "let's."
   e. Use stories or anecdotes.
   f. Remember that words like "right" and "truth" put you on the positive side of any debate.
   g. Know when to be silent.

6. Problem-Solving Process:
   a. Clearly identify the problem/task.
   b. Review available resources.
   c. Select alternatives for this situation.
   d. Write a Plan A and Plan B.
   e. Establish measurements of success.
   f. Implement the plan—take action!
   g. Evaluate outcomes.

CHAPTER FOUR

Inside Finishing

Sharing the Vision and Power with Others

Having lost sight of our objective, we redoubled our efforts.

Continuous Quality Improvement

The pursuit of quality ... the ability to practice at the level of medical and surgical care that is state of the art ... the desire for service excellence. These are the objectives of most veterinarians in practice today. Most practices want the staff to deliver quality healthcare at all times—continuous quality care. The disappointing fact that escapes the average practitioner is that "quality" is an outcome of the healthcare delivery system, not just a single element of the input. It cannot be mandated; it must be perceived by the client. The client perceives pride; pride is a critical indicator of quality care.

Total quality management (TQM), as promoted and implemented for American industry by noted authors/consultants such as Joe Juran, Ed Deming, or Phil Crosby, does not often translate directly to American healthcare delivery, and especially not directly to veterinary healthcare delivery. Quality in veterinary practice is a perception of the client, based most often on communication and events not of a veterinary technical manner. There are technical elements as well as service elements that affect the client's perception, which is why a continuous quality improvement (CQI) system must be implemented at all levels of a veterinary practice.

The *L* in Quality Stands for Leadership

The traditional approach to quality emphasized evaluating the symptoms and implementing a low-cost quick fix to ensure the symptoms did not recur. This was called quality assurance—an after-action, spot-check system. Although this approach far better than nothing, permanent changes were rare because root causes were seldom identified or solved. In healthcare marketing, quality isn't an internal definition—it is an external perception, a total caring cycle with continuous improvements. The best quality results when the provider accepts the idea that "It is my reputation," when teamwork breaks down barriers to allow shared prevention, and when all staff members accept the value of striving to exceed client and practice expectations.

QA Versus CQI

Quality assurance (QA) has traditionally been an internal focus on spot-checking past events. Continuous quality improvement requires the focus to be divided among three areas: external, internal, and self. Quality assurance leads to reactive management and casting blame, whereas CQI lends itself to establishing precedence, policy, procedure, and processes to meet the goals. Quality assurance reinforces the need for supervisory control (top-down management), whereas CQI must be based on prevention of quality slippage (team environment). QA promotes an adversarial climate, whereas CQI promotes harmony and cooperation. Quality assurance forces a vertical line of control in a practice, whereas CQI promotes a horizontal system of practice management.

Quality is defined at multiple levels. Clients will define it based on expectations, desires, preferences, and the way their needs are noticed and addressed. Veterinarians will define it based on the techniques that reflect levels of care similar to the training occurring in universities and continuing education. The paraprofessional staff will often define it based on perceptions of caring and empathy, as well as comparisons to other practices in the community. Suppliers/vendors will base their evaluation of quality upon the equipment and supplies being procured and brought to bear on the diagnostics and healthcare implementation plan.

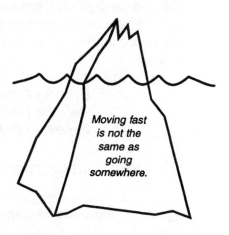

Moving fast is not the same as going somewhere.

Pride Is the Input

The traditional approach that quality is dictated by management has not been an effective method to ensure quality in healthcare. If we accept the concept that quality is an outcome, a perception of others, then the input must be a factor that affects all delivery and client communications. That common factor is pride.

Pride is the self-dictated task of exceeding expectations. It is never asking, "Why didn't somebody do it?" but rather, "Why didn't I see it occurring and do something?" The traditional reliance on the job descriptions that were so popular in the 1980s destroyed the zest for the quest. The use of core values for managers and a list of critical accountability areas for each individual has been most successful to promote pride in exceeding expectations. At one hospital, "pride" was redefined as "core values" by replacing the letters with words:

Patient   The patient always comes first ... and first, do no harm.
Respect   Mutual respect among the team, and consideration for the
             client and the patient, are primary.
Innovation   Each employee was hired to solve problems, not just to
             do a job.
Dedication   The quality outcome of every encounter should be every-
             one's goal.
Excellence   Competency is the best possible performance.

Every member of the staff must realize that he or she was hired not merely to do a job, but to solve problems. Practice is a series of problems, to be prevented, solved, or minimized. The problem with hands-on management is what occurs when you take the hands away. It is one reason participative management often fails in a healthcare delivery system. To lead is to set boundaries, expect certain outcomes, and develop measurements for that outcome. Peter Drucker's MBWA (management by walking around) has become altered to management by walking away. Allowing staff members to thrash around and learn more about the alternatives can be a building experience to increase effectiveness in future behavior, especially if followed by face-to-face dialogue. Behavior can be a protection or a projection of self, and your management style will make the staff member select the one needed to survive in the practice environment.

Because I dissent, I am not disloyal ...
Because I differ, I am not disloyal ...
Because I care, I will challenge assumptions.

Change Management

To make change happen, three ingredients are needed in your management approach: determination, education, and implementation. The real determination originates from dissatisfaction with the present, and from your helping the staff recognize that action is the only tool available to effect change. Staff education is more than just exploring the alternatives to a difficult situation; it is helping all staff members learn a common practice behavior based on quality, personal accountability, and pride. Implementation is the repetition of the behavior until the pursuit of higher quality becomes new habit—a pursuit that is never quite finished because we keep seeing what can be (CQI). But each step increases the health of the practice.

In many cases continuous quality improvement is perceived as the elimination of hassles. Our research has shown that the most common hassle for the staff is the demotivation that occurs in most practices. The leadership's response to inquiries and suggestions cause the staff's innovation and dedication to dry up.

We hire staff members because they impress us, they meet our needs, and they have strengths that we appreciate. I don't know of any practice that hires because of incompetency, bad attitudes, or weaknesses. In some practices the drive for excellence and improvement is killed by phrases like: "We don't do it that way here," "Don't make waves," or "As the new person, you have to learn our ways or leave." As general malaise sets in, to assist in survival, the practice owner starts to talk about the need for better communication and teamwork. This is usually a genuine effort to improve the work environment; a search is initiated for the quick fix, the consultant with the guaranteed answer, or the book that tells it all.

In the 1980s veterinary practice management saw the increase of detailed job descriptions, policy manuals, and retrospective performance appraisals. There were very few people trained and certified as effective reviewers, especially in veterinary medicine. In human healthcare the hospitals saw participative management come and go. Seems the doctors didn't want the team to decide how patient care was to be prescribed, and the disease-related groups (DRGs) of the third-party payers could wait for a decision. In industry, quality circles and strategic planning were passing cures (or curses, if you actually had to try working within one of these top-level brainstorms). The advent of staff meetings provided a great place for the important people to hear themselves talk, but seldom caused any system changes. The role of faithful listener falls on the majority, and the role of decision maker usually is held by someone other than the person doing the daily task.

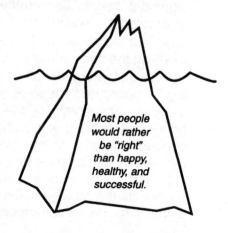

Most people would rather be "right" than happy, healthy, and successful.

Life has some built-in hassles, but we bring those upon ourselves. In a practice hassles can be prevented—not item by item, but by communicating both ways. Hassled people do not pursue quality work. A hassle is when the staff or boss spends more time working on each other than on making something happen for the client or patient. A hassle-free environment is one where any staff member can use the core values of the practice to make life better for a client or patient, without having to get permission from anyone or worry about consequences. This staff member empowerment is a step toward the continuous quality improvement (CQI), but it must be nurtured.

The Truths

In developing an action plan to confront the habits that a practice needs to change to advance into CQI, there are five truths that must be accepted:

1. There is no more time in any day.

2. Quality occurs after expectations are met.

3. Prevention will lead to quality.

4. Fear of failure prevents quality growth and change.

5. Nonconformity is the price of quality.

A continuous quality improvement environment is built by getting everyone to do it right the first time (Phil Crosby calls this DIRFT). The key to DIRFT lies with the hospital director establishing clear expectations, assigning accountabilities rather than tasks, and not accepting any excuses or problems. Time is saved when each person accepts the responsibility (and has the authority) to make client-centered decisions unilaterally, just by using the core values of the practitioner and the practice. Hassle results when a staff member knows what needs to be done but must kill time waiting for approval from someone else. In DIRFT "it" is the requirement, the assigned accountability, the latitude, to make a decision and implement new ideas without worry about management approval. Honda took this concept one step further by requiring every employee idea to be implemented by management for 90 days before it was evaluated.

If we produce widgets, there is a quality control team that ensures every widget fits the prototype. If it does not, they assign blame and require that a quick fix be implemented. In a service industry like healthcare, it is harder to evaluate restoration of wellness. This is especially true when the veterinary schools teach only maintenance of wellness. The secret of CQI lies in the prevention of hassles. Each practice must look at every process and identify the opportunities for error. These can be controlled. Every service a veterinary practice provides contains many components managed by multiple people; each element must be dealt with individually to eliminate the potential cause(s) of any problem. CQI is based on constant evaluation and feedback from staff and clients to allow better assessment of potential problems.

The fear of failure often means that repetition becomes the standard. If we do what we did yesterday because we didn't get into trouble, then we won't have to worry ... except that the lack of change is stasis, and stasis, in healthcare is another term for death. Metafane was replaced by halothane, which is being replaced by isofluorane, which will likely be replaced by the end of the decade ... but there are still practices using metafane. There are still practices not using X rays or ECGs in routine diagnostics. Neither metafane nor ECGs are client or patient centered. Healthcare is an art and a science; given this reality, mistakes will occur, but they should be restricted to those times we try new things. Making first mistakes means we are making discoveries while learning; repeating mistakes means we didn't learn. Establishing performance standards, measurements that can be seen and accomplished, is the key to controlling the direction and intensity of errors. If you can't measure it, you can't manage it.

Errors cost money. Failure to conform to standards costs money. However, the inverse is not always true: the absence of errors does not mean that the practice is making more money. Conformity is necessary to an extent, but it, too, has a cost. Conformity means attention to the process, and attention to the process will ingrain both good and bad habits. As a practice grows, established habits must be changed; non-conformity to community-accepted procedures will occur and is desirable. The practice that keeps the cost of this nonconformity within reason will be the one that produces new outcomes that differentiate it in the community marketplace at an economically profitable level of operation. Educating the staff to techniques of innovation will cause growth faster than training staff to follow the process that the boss has established. Transfer of understanding is the true education. The understanding of why, the belief in the core values of the practice, and

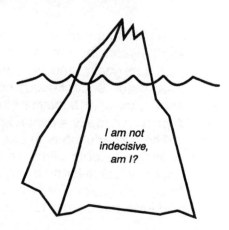

I am not indecisive, am I?

the understanding of the practice goals for the year, as well as the long-range planning concerns, will be the elements that control the level of non-conformity while leading to continuous quality improvement.

The L Factor

The organizational champion is the leader, the person who believes in the strength of the individual. Leaders must have followers, but managers need only projects. Leaders will be the answer to survive the chaos of the 1990s predicted by futurist Tom Peters. What CQI requires is a leader who incorporates service excellence and caring into daily activities. There are six leadership principles that apply to the CQI program:

1. Preach and lead with vision—without it, your staff will lack direction and inspiration.

2. Always practice what you preach, set the standard and the example— your actions speak far louder than your words.

3. Make people accountable—encourage your team members to have pride in the outcomes, not in adherence to a process.

4. Empower your staff—support them, ask, listen, inform, act, recognize, and reward; create heroes and superstars.

5. Take risks—stick your neck out; opportunity and danger are inseparable. Trigger change, don't direct it.

6. Go for the long haul, not the quick fix—don't start a plan unless you have the energy to follow up; commit the dollars, invest in continuous quality improvement.

Management philosophy and commitment set the stage and enable the key players, the practice staff, to move in the same direction, reach for common goals, and be measured by fair standards. By starting with a clear vision of continuous quality improvement in service excellence, you set the tone for behavior standards. We can affect behavior, not attitude. A poor attitude is a symptom, not a cause.

The leader's job is to build a responsive healthcare delivery team—responsive to both client and patient needs. The leader initiates this responsive behavior by being responsive to the staff's needs. Leaders need to communicate clearly and openly to build understanding, commitment, and investment, and to enforce and reinforce inviolable high personal values leading to equally high performance standards. With the management commitment to CQI, you can have a value-driven practice that has strength, focus, and inspiration at the delivery level as well as at the helm. CQI is a philosophy, a multiyear program of effort and retraining. It is not the quick fix of yesterday. When staff start to resist, begin to doubt your judgment in attempting to bring about change, or in wishing for the good old days. Remember the following quote:

> *The significant problems that we face today*
> *cannot be solved at the same level of thinking that created them.*
> —Albert Einstein

The Pillars of CQI Excellence

If you want quality to be a perceived outcome,

then pride must be the input!

The last sentence of the hiring interview is important, and mine is, "If you don't like to sweat, don't take the job!" Once the person has accepted the job offer, the last sentence of the hiring action can set the tone for the rest of the employment. I also like to say, "Remember that job description we discussed—well, forget it; you are not being hired to do a job, you are joining this team to help solve problems!"

The reality of continuous quality improvement (CQI) is that it can't be a one-shot program. Participative management training is the beginning of the concept, but CQI goes beyond that level of team building. In participative management the team is built around goals and objectives of the leader. In CQI the programs and processes are built around the vision of the person doing the job. Tomorrow will be better than today; next month we will do it better than last month; six months from now you will see major changes; one year from now you won't recognize the operation—then we start for another plane of excellence.

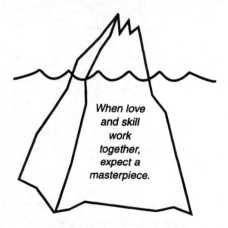

When love and skill work together, expect a masterpiece.

Talking about the pride of ownership or

the clear empowerment of the individual is simple to do, but the concepts must be built on a foundation of solid principles. The guiding skills of the foundation, of long-term support system development, can be called the pillars of CQI excellence. When planning the architecture of any new construction, the hidden foundation will allow it to withstand the test of time and the tremors of impending disaster. Each piling or pillar represents a powerful force that must stand solid and supportive and yet, in conjunction with the others, point in the same direction to support the CQI, and to service a program of excellence. The continuous quality care foundation of the healthcare delivery system rests on 10 pillars (see Figure 4.1).

Trust in Values

That the first pillar of CQI includes the words "trust" and "values" is not an accident. The staff member's trust in values is critical to his or her continuous quality improvement efforts. The core values of the practice, the attending veterinarian, and management must be consistent and predictable. When someone makes an operational decision based on the core values of the practice, that person needs to know he or she will be supported and even complimented, not attacked, regardless of the outcome. The core values must not be difficult to remember or overdefined. McDonald's uses Q-S-V-C (clients *always* deserve, and want: quality, service, value, cleanliness). There is one human hospital that uses PRIDE to remind everyone of the five factors: "patient," "respect," "innovation," "dedication," and "excellence." As practice consultants, we have used I CARE:

T	C	A	R	T	C	R	E	E	P
R	O	C	E	R	O	E	X	V	R
U	M	C	C	A	M	M	P	A	O
S	M	O	O	I	M	I	E	L	B
T	I	U	G	N	U	N	C	U	L
	T	N	N	I	N	D	T	A	E
I	M	T	I	N	I	E	A	T	M
N	E	A	T	G	C	R	T	I	
	N	B	I		A	S	I	O	S
V	T	I	O		T		O	N	O
A		L	N		I		N		L
L		I			O		S		V
U		T			N				I
E		Y							N
S									G

Fig. 4.1. The ten pillars of CQI

- Clients ... they always come first;
- Action ... clients and staff want this;
- Respect ... for yourself, the client, the patient, and the team;
- Excellence ... competency is expected;
- and I ... because that is who can make the difference.

Commitment

Continuous quality improvement and service excellence are not just programs. The commitment must become an organization value, and it must be pervasive at every level of operation. Employees, especially healthcare employees, need to identify with an organization that strives to exemplify values and standards they believe in. This commitment motivates and inspires when management exemplifies the commitment. The CQI practice can never allow itself to become a "Do-what-I-say, not-what-I-do" environment. This commitment promotes openness, and the willingness to take risks, and rests on the working assumption that client perceptions reflect reality.

Accountability

The practice delegates or assigns accountabilities, never tasks; accountabilities are monitored for end results, not for the process. Job descriptions should assign areas of responsibility and accountability, with clear quality and service standards that can be measured. Are the expected behaviors well defined, or are vague terms like "attitude" and "human relations" used to obscure the expectations? Explicit expectations, using the right person for the right job, and developing a formal commendation system for achievement are critical elements to ensure that continuous quality improvement accountability is promoted and nurtured.

Recognition

The fourth pillar does not need to be in a special position within the foundation of CQI. In fact, recognition is one CQI pillar that requires innovation and multiple applications to become an effective tool. Excellence may be its own reward, but it is better to assume that it isn't. Part of the CQI strategy is to reward that behavior which needs to be repeated, and to starve that which needs to be lost and forgotten. Exemplary energy, behavior, or a sense of commitment needs recogni-

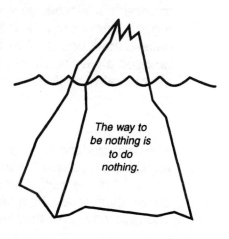

The way to be nothing is to do nothing.

tion and reward on a regular basis; please do not restrict recognition to task accomplishment. The traditional "employee of the month" program makes most of the staff losers, unless the award is reduced to a "sequential turn" program. Look for people who buy into the CQI concept, and reward small feats, minor miracles, or other demonstrations of pride, excellence, or commitment to the practice values.

Training

The fifth pillar of continuous quality improvement helps people sharpen their commonsense skills in the arts of meeting, greeting, and performing. Job titles do not bestow job knowledge or the required understanding of new expectations and quality standards. Invest time, money, and personal concern in the training and retraining of practice staff members to make CQI a personal capability.

Communication

This CQI pillar is not a polite cop-out. It is a commitment to force downward information flow and to promote upward and lateral evaluation and feedback. Employee attitude surveys have proven that staff morale is defeated more by no news than by bad news. The ability to give *and* get information, not just data, makes for an effective CQI communication standard.

Reminders

The seventh pillar means more than sending postcards to clients about vaccinations. As time passes, awareness fades. A host of other problems clutter the already overworked minds of the practice staff. The leader must take action to remind the staff that continuous quality improvement and service excellence are still important to their mind-set and approaches. In practice, we are always in competition for a staff member's attention, so you have to consciously institute methods that trigger attention to CQI. If the leader does not do this, staff members will believe that because their hearts are in the right place, their habits must be good also. The rituals that revive awareness and commitment must be innovative and targeted to command the undivided attention of the staff.

Expectations

The expectations pillar is a unique component of continuous quality improvement because it means multiple things, depending on one's point of view. For the basic CQI concept, it means that tomorrow will be made better than today because staff members are empowered to make changes whenever they see a need to improve client or patient care. To the leadership it means that the standards must be clear, that taking risks and sharing the truth will be promoted and rewarded. To the team it means the expectation of a satisfied and productive workplace where they are understood, nurtured, and happy.

Evaluation

The CQI pillar of evaluation goes beyond communication. Evaluation occurs when the information flow becomes knowledge and that knowledge is used to promote change. This pillar centers on gathering information from clients, staff, and the community, then using that information to guide the planning for tomorrow. With the concept of continuous quality improvement you cannot navigate blindly; you must strive to meet needs in a better manner. You must always be ready to be enlightened by someone else.

Problem Solving

Last, but not least, of the 10 pillars is problem solving, but it could just as easily be termed complaint management or innovation promotion. It is the charter for every member of the staff to access system problems, practice challenges, or just the minor nagging frustrations that reduce the daily quality of life. Each of the other pillars depends on this pillar strengthening the foundation of the continuous quality improvement efforts. This pillar brings to mind the initial premise of employment, which is: "You were not hired to do a job; you were hired to solve problems."

Strong Pillars Make for Strong Practices

As you now realize, these pillars are not sequential or chronological. You may choose to start building at any point. You cannot ignore any of the pillars, because together they form the unity of the foundation. If you believe that the practice offers a high level of quality, review the staff's level of pride. If pride is high, quality will be high, but pride will not always lead to the changes needed to meet the emerging demands of the pet-owning community.

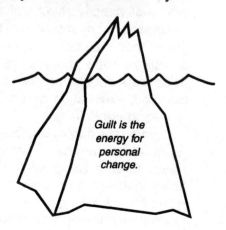

Guilt is the energy for personal change.

Change occurs because of dissatisfaction with the current situation. If you hear constant rationalization or defensive comments, expert the status quo to be maintained. Remember, yesterday's quality procedure is common in today's average practice. As you review these concepts, either here or in the current best-selling texts about quality by authors like J.M. Juran, Philip B. Crosby, or W. Edwards Deming, let this new philosophy catapult you forward in planning a comprehensive and well-supported strategy for implementing CQI in your practice.

The Only Constant Is Change

What we have learned in most of the 800 veterinary facilities we have visited in the past three years is one simple idea: "We don't know where we are or where we are going, but quite clearly, we are getting there awfully fast." Many veterinary practices sprinted through the rapid growth of the 1970s and capitalized on the vaccination of parvo puppies in the early 1980s. Most have started to encounter the traumatic cutbacks caused by increased densities of veterinarians in their area, increased client awareness, and the infusion of healthcare substitutes by pet stores and humane societies. In the 1980s young people quit pursuing secure healthcare careers to follow the lure of investment banking, high-rolling law firms, and other yuppie pursuits. These trendy careers are now overwhelmed with anxiety and disappointment, and university admission applications for healthcare careers are increasing again. Change is a constant.

A systems approach to managing change is a must if long-term benefits are expected to result. All of the influencing factors (leaders and staff members) must push in the same direction, or the staff gets confused. This means the practice philosophy, value system, and mission statement must be taught by example. If a practice owner says one thing and does another as a leader, the messages on the walls will become a joke, as will other practice goals. The consistency of behavior of managers and staff, the scope and frequency of skill building, the nature of job expectations, hiring practices, communication systems, and training and retraining programs all directly affect staff behavior and client perceptions and must be integrated. If any member of the staff is allowed to ignore these integrated goals, then they become voluntary rather than expected. If they are not integrated—if the practice system endorses conflicting values or behavior, or delivers double messages—staff members are thrown into an impossible bind. Frustration and burnout develop, and employees become angry—and rightfully so!

Continuous quality improvement (CQI) is an ongoing process, not a program. A program has a beginning and an end—it is a discrete event. CQI needs to be a value within the performance expectations. It needs to be firmly installed, then actively and aggressively maintained forever: recognition for risk taking rather than risk avoidance needs to be pursued in an innovative manner. This requires a culture change in most veterinary practices. Organizational change has three steps, as described by behavioral scientist Kurt Lewis:

- UNFREEZING—thawing out established behavior patterns
- CHANGING—moving to a new behavior pattern
- REFREEZING—maintaining the new pattern

To make these steps occur, you need a long-term plan with short-term goals and objectives, as well as clear intermediate expectations. It will not be easy; it will take courage; but it will also be worth the effort because of the rewards and continuity of care that thoughtful planning promotes.

Three-Stage Planning Process

There have been many customer relations programs that were a great disappointment. Also, a client-centered orientation hasn't always produced the desired results. Most of these disasters occurred because programs and efforts were launched before the practice was ready; they failed because of impatience. Eagerness and excitement about promises and possibilities does not make a program successful. Meticulous, comprehensive, and thoughtful deliberation by the entire healthcare delivery team is required.

You need to make the practice foundation strong before constructing the edifice itself. The goal of planning is to ensure that your strategy is carefully tailored to fit your practice's current realities and its problems, culture, and staff. If you have no strategy yet, or if you feel the need to regroup or regenerate a better approach, institute a three-stage CQI planning process before you enter the task-planning process of Chapter 3:

STAGE 1 TAKE THE TPR OF YOUR PRACTICE. What is your competitive position, image, culture, and norms? Also, what is the status of practice pride and perceived quality?

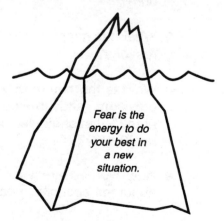

Fear is the energy to do your best in a new situation.

STAGE 2 CHARACTERIZE YOUR STAFF. Identify the segments or subgroups within your practice, their concept of success, their dreams and personal desires.

STAGE 3 IDENTIFY COMPONENTS OF A BEST-FIT STRATEGY.
Ensure that you address the needs and concerns of every staff member.
Motivate each group and take steps to anticipate and minimize resistance.

This all sounds simple enough for the experienced practitioner who has
the time and skill to develop a long-term, innovative process like continuous quality improvement. But, then, this does not describe the average
veterinary practitioner who is stretched to the limit for time, effort, and ability to handle the crisis of the moment. Here are some TPR questions that
must be asked before starting any CQI process:

- Exactly where is the income compared to the same period last year?
  Where are the finances really going? What are the seasonal versus
  community trends?

- How serious is the liquidity problem? What is the real profit-and-loss
  picture for the previous 24 months?

- What are the population and economic trends affecting your practice? What has happened to the number of new clients per month,
  and how many have been acquired by referrals from other clients?

- What are the trends for transactions, in real numbers as well as in the
  average client transaction? Are clients coming in more or less frequently? What is the overhead expense trend per client transaction?

- What kind of patients do you have? Does the mix match the community and national trend for type of pet ownership? What are the
  trends of inpatient versus outpatient user, and expense per procedure?

- What has happened to the accounts-receivable trends, and for what
  reasons?

- What is the nature of your competition? Who are the new and old
  providers, and how do they impact upon the practice catchment
  area? What strategies do they use, and who is winning (by what values)? Why?

- How worried are your staff, the veterinarians, and their spouses
  about the economic health of the practice?

■ How does the pet-owning public perceive your practice and your competitors? What kind of reputation does your practice have in the community? How have you determined that the assumptions you make are valid?

■ How do colleagues perceive your healthcare delivery standards and capabilities? How do they rate your services and staff?

■ What are are recurring complaints from clients, staff, vendors, and visitors? How do the various users of your services characterize the behavior of your workforce?

■ What are the prevailing attitudes of staff toward one another, the work environment, the clients and patients, and their own jobs?

■ How have staff members responded in the past to problem solving? How have they participated to better the practice, the healthcare delivery, or the quality of employee life?

■ How do your staff perceive resistance to change, from themselves, veterinarians, owners, spouses, clients, and the community in general?

■ How much do your people trust one another? What is the level of respect between professionals and paraprofessionals? Is there a difference, and why?

■ How do your staff feel about working here? Is productivity high or low? Do they they can influence performance or productivity standards?

■ How good is the boss's understanding of the day-to-day hassles of the job? Has the manager ever performed the job for a period of time to experience its operational challenges?

■ How regular is the communication process for nonmedical issues? Does everyone know the practice goals for this year? This month? How often are opinions and feelings elicited and

A great many people think they are thinking when they are merely rearranging their prejudices.

acted upon? How often are the staff provided updates on practice trends and programs?

■ How often are morale-boosting events held? Who attends? Who gets to plan them? Who evaluates them after the event?

■ To what extent do people smile and joke? How is talking promoted or curtailed between staff members? How often are impassive faces experienced or tolerated? What is the definition of "professional behavior" within the different elements of the practice team?

■ How much pride do people take in their work space? What personal effects are allowed in their work space to assist in their feeling of ownership? How do staff present themselves, in appearance and posture?

■ How proud are your people of the healthcare traditions that they support? Do they access care for their own pets? How well do the different groups cooperate or carp?

■ How often do people take the initiative? How often do you hear "That's not my job," or "I am too busy to help you"? How many times does the phone ring before a technician will answer it? Before a veterinarian will answer it?

■ How much cooperation occurs between shifts? Between staff groups? How often does the practice ask for a second opinion from a respected colleague? How often are referrals used to increase the quality of care offered?

■ When was the last staff meeting held? When was the last client survey? How was the information gathered used? Who conducts the exit interview with departing clients, and what is the nature of the feedback? What happens to suggestions or comments?

As we determine the practice TPR, new ideas will evolve. Habits will emerge, as will frustrations. Change will be seen either as progressive or as a disaster. When you characterize the staff, there is a series of questions you can ask to validate the TPR discoveries or to expand on the information at hand:

■ How does the receptionist team behave toward clients who enter or depart the reception area? How do they deal with telephone shoppers?

- Who sets the dress standard? Who sets the behavior standard? What are the existing dress and behavior standards? (They do exist, whether stated or not.)

- How do the animal caretakers characterize the practice? How do the maintenance staff characterize the practice? Do the paraprofessional support staff characterize the practice in the same terms as the clients do?

- What attitudinal predispositions are common among the receptionist team? The technician team? The caretaker team? Between the veterinarians? The spouses? Where did the attitude originate?

- When the receptionist staff are confronted with the idea of change, how do they react? How do the technician staff respond? What does the owner do when confronted with a need for change, or with a request?

- What are the major obstacles to change in the practice? Do the different staff groups perceive the same obstacles?

When you have taken stock of the organizational climate and the practice's competitive position in the community, you need to reconsider the attitudes, values, and behavior of target populations as well as of the staff. This information will allow the practice to develop a sound strategy based on information and knowledge. When you design the CQI strategy, a best-fit process can be developed internally or with the help of a facilitator, but it must affect the heterogeneous client and staff groups concurrently. It is sad, but we cannot hold a workshop for cynics one day and enthusiasts the next day. We can't hold a selective charm school to fit client to staff. Each staff member has different feelings and perspectives, and your strategy needs to speak to all of these effectively. The situation is not easy because what works to motivate one person runs the risk of alienating others.

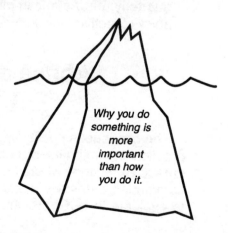

Why you do something is more important than how you do it.

If all staff members, as well as leadership, were willing and able, life would be easy. But life is diverse, and we find the willing and unable, the cooperative but distracted, the resigned, the oppressed, the resentful, the cynics, the rebellious, and the insulted within our team. And people aren't the same every day. You can't change attitudes, but you can require behavior change. The components of a best-fit strategy start with this concept.

As a final word of warning in building the CQI process upon the pillars we have discussed, please keep in mind the following:

Beware of Flashes in the Pan
Do not go for short-term enthusiasm, especially if you have a "this too shall pass" history of idea implementation. Build on a solid foundation of principles and values.

Start by Clarifying Your Vision
Know where you are and be sure you know exactly where you want to go. Do not distract the team by frequently changing your vision.

Involve a Wide Array of Key People from the Start
Total staff buy-in starts with the planning process. CQI plans are worthless unless the staff participate in the development. The power of the planning process lies in the commitment of the participants, the clarity of purpose, and the sense of a common direction. Cooperation is the key to making things happen.

Make CQI a Lifetime Commitment for the Practice
The value of the process lies in the promise of a better tomorrow, a vision that anyone can impact with personal effort. To renew staff motivation, you will need to conduct an active evaluation process monthly and quarterly; the American mind does not usually set achievable (measurable) objectives for periods over 90 days.

Abuse and Neglect of the CQI Process

The continuous quality improvement process is based on the long-term practice commitment of establishing pride and empowering the staff to pursue excellence wherever the need is identified. Abuse and neglect are companion terms; we use them in animal welfare and can also use them to evaluate the CQI process; abuse requires proving intent, whereas neglect simply evaluates the outcomes. As with most long-term operations, the lapse of time dulls the intensity of emphasis. Although most quality practices that adopt CQI as a cornerstone will not abuse the CQI principles, neglect can creep into the operation. This may be due to multiple factors, but the most common is that entrenched habits of the past resurface when leadership fails to maintain focus.

Shake Up Your System

The following are common entrenched habits that must be shaken at the roots, then recalibrated, for the process of continuous quality improvement to be accepted as an emerging practice value.

Emphasis on short-term profits. Americans want immediate gratification, whether it be fast food or easy practice management techniques. The current trend to control expenses to make profit can work only in practices that are managed poorly. The profit increases from cost control do not make the money pie bigger; they only give you a bigger piece at this sitting. Well-managed practices already have cost-control procedures and need to consider long-term income programs. This means an investment of time and money, usually longer periods of time for the transition than ever needed before in the practice. Long-term programs need to be considered carefully because equipment, training, and client education will usually be required to make them consistently profitable.

Management by fear. The traditional performance evaluation promotes short-term performance at the expense of long-term planning; it discourages risk taking, pits people against each other for common rewards, and undermines the teamwork required to improve practice performance. The insidious effect is an increased reliance on arbitrary merit pay numbers rather than on team performance. Some veterinarians dread making judgments of their staff; CQI is an answer to this fear. Competition is not required for excellence, as demonstrated by historical figures like Einstein, Bach, or Shakespeare. People work for themselves far better than they work for an employer. The job of a leader is to reduce limitations and to increase the capabilities of the people he or she influences.

Observation is the key to transformation.

Decisions based on numbers alone. The

use of easy-to-get figures is a starting point for management, as are participative management techniques for the staff. But continuous quality improvement requires a stretch beyond these established habits. The effect of a happy client on new client referrals is hard to measure and greatly variable, but it is critical to success in an overpopulated veterinary healthcare community. The value of effective communication and problem resolution is impossible to measure, unless it goes astray. Pride can make a difference, but there are no numbers that reflect the pride in performance that a staff member feels after a hard day at the practice grind.

Inability to accept change. The good news of CQI must be preceded by the bad news that something is wrong. The discomfort of accepting this fact should be cause for changing habits, not for changing practice staff. The person elevating a problem to the level of attempting a solution is to be commended, not chastised and defined out of existence. A change strategy is based on the identification of a problem, a frustration, or a distraction, and the developing dissatisfaction and discomfort that accompanies the discovery. This discomfort should lead to the evaluation of alternatives to reach new goals and objectives, the systematic education and training of all staff involved, the implementation and evaluation of a test plan, and, finally, the leadership action necessary to establish new habits among the practice staff and within the daily operations.

Lack of constancy. The privilege of the practice owner to state a set of rules and procedures, then grant exceptions, is an American right. It is also a reason that American management has been by-passed by emerging industrial countries. If the staff cannot trust ownership to support their decisions, they will not make workmanship decisions; they will play it safe. Dedication to the principles of CQI must be widespread, constant, and promoted on a regular basis. It is not enough just to announce the CQI commitment, because all employees have seen great ideas come and go during the life of a practice; they need proof. One way is money—money for training and equipment, or for stopping an operational process that violates CQI values. The leadership must take time to explain and discuss the CQI process in full.

Neglect of long-range planning. Even with a clear and achievable long-range plan, practices get derailed because of personnel problems, economic recessions, or other emergencies not in the plan. Many times the principles of CQI are forgotten because of frivolous attention to insignificant details, such as someone who left early one day because his or her work was done. If pride in performance and outcome is present, is it really important when the minutes tick off the time clock? When pursuing continuous quality improvement, a good leader will not get lost in the trivia of past parameters but, rather, will set new team goals that elicit a move toward greatness and pride.

Adding toys instead of commitment. The addition of a new endoscope does not increase staff commitment to continuous quality improvement, although it is something to boast about at the local VMA meeting. A new dental base or new anesthesia machine does not convey concern for a client's needs; that is done by staff members on a regular basis, by phone, at the reception desk, in the exam room, or out in the community. Equipment is secondary to the healthcare delivery commitment of a dedicated team.

Blaming others for problems. Too often a practitioner blames the environment, the competition, or even the staff for problems. The simple fact is that only 15 percent of problems are influenced by the staff of a healthcare facility; the other 85 percent are due to the system or management of the system. Quality control and quality assurance are based on discovering errors, assigning blame, and establishing a quick fix. CQI is based on responding to change before it occurs by making habits and procedures more responsive to the emerging demands of clients, staff, and healthcare providers.

Defining quality too narrowly. If the end result of CQI is defined in terms of healthcare services and technological advancements, the staff begin to see themselves as secondary to the effort. If a leader stresses that no person is too low in the organization to be excluded, and no person is too privileged to be exempt from evaluation and change, he or she has found the winning secret for continuous quality improvement. The definition of quality must include clinical outcome, service to the client, management structure, staff process, and pride in the process at every level of the practice.

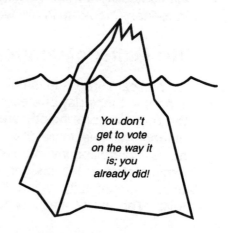

You don't get to vote on the way it is; you already did!

In Practice

To consider anything less than quality performance in healthcare seems unthinkable. Quality has always been an explicit goal in veterinary medicine, so why is it being rediscovered? Why do clients price shop, and why do colleagues offer discounts, if quality is explicit? The answer is attitude versus behavior, theory versus reality, rhetoric versus action. Managers do things right; leaders do the right things.

Continuous quality improvement is not just something the veterinarian buys into to improve quality or productivity, although these are outcomes of the process. CQI is a way of life that must be lived consistently, day by day. The ownership must "walk the talk" of organizational values and purpose. Genuine leaders create, embody, and communicate the vision, values, and sense of mission needed to establish pride in the practice. There are no shortcuts to developing continuous quality improvement as a practice process for the 1990s. Everyone must just do it!

Quality Transformation

Quality—in its classic Greek sense: how to live with grace and intelligence, with bravery and mercy, with humble pride.

Quality transformation in any organization takes time. Total quality management was introduced by W. Edwards Deming in Japan because the American industrial system was not ready for it. J.M. Juran was able to introduce TQM into the production-line American industries because Japan had "stolen" the market, and Philip Crosby carried TQM into white-collar America because it worked at other levels of business. The lateral TQM movement in healthcare was slower yet, until healthcare providers got into continuous quality improvement. CQI did not require buy-in from the physicians to work; it needed only a caring and dedicated leader (hospital administrator) who was willing to release control, and a staff willing to accept accountability for the outcomes to accomplish the improvement process. Veterinary medicine is still waiting to start.

The Matter of Control

The licensure issue is not the problem in releasing control; the problem is habits. Since day one every veterinarian has been held accountable for the outcome of a healthcare delivery episode. This will not change. But management is more than healthcare episodes. It is scheduling staff hours, controlling inventories, promoting the practice, solving client problems, watching the budget, managing the staff, standardizing protocols, ensuring continuity of care in multidoctor facilities, and a host of administrivia. The list of ancillary functions seems endless, and will be unless everyone in the practice becomes accountable for better outcomes of daily activities.

Start at the front desk: who makes the decision on the new appointment log format? In most cases the doctor, but the reception team could really make a format more applicable and easier to use. Moving further back into the practice flow, who does the wellness screening physical on vaccination appointments? Usually the doctor, but a trained technician could do it and expedite the process before the doctor even arrives. Who monitors the expiration dates of drugs, especially controlled substances? Usually no one! A trained staff member could easily accept this drug-monitoring function. Who does the client callbacks after surgery? A staff member could, but usually the doctor doesn't have time, so it doesn't get done! Who makes the bank deposits? Who schedules the staff? Who manages the pet boarding and grooming scheduling to ensure that a consolidated and full schedule is maintained? Who ensures that the handouts and flyers are kept current and client friendly? In most hospitals the answer to these questions is the same: "When the doctor gets time." Yet staff can do it all.

The staff must be properly taught, if the life of the practice is to be extended. This will require a change in the habits, in the paradigms, of the owner and veterinarians. It will require each to release control of the process, to help others accept accountability for the end results, and to shift emphasis from process to outcome. It will require an uncommon leadership willing to commit to continuous change and improvement.

The uncommon leader is one who understands that CQI is a commitment to a new process, a process controlled by the staff. The staff can see what needs to be done; they must now accept accountability for making the changes happen. They need to be protected from unexpected lightning bolts—from the limitations of the past. The "Why did you do that?" must be replaced by an understanding of the caring intentions and well-meaning efforts of every staff member. The final quality and release of control associated with results-oriented activities is based on understanding the CQI cycle and the essential steps of the planning process outlined in Chapter 3 (see Figure 4.2).

Planning starts by defining the desired outcome, then defining the outcome within the available system(s). The staff member knows best which pressures cause the distractions. The discussion may need leadership support and encouragement, as having unilateral accountability for change may

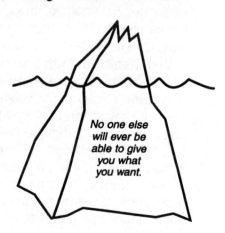

No one else will ever be able to give you what you want.

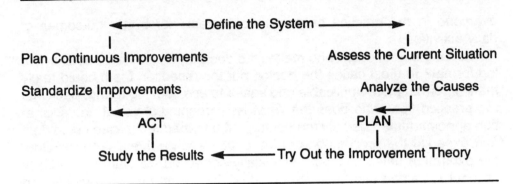

Fig. 4.2. The CQI cycle

well be a new concept. The system may first seem expansive, but joint discussions can pare it down to bite-sized projects (90-day activities). When the current situation is assessed, all the available resources must be evaluated, including time, people, money, and motivation. As the causes are assessed, care should be taken not to allocate blame but, rather, to seek future prevention and acceptable alternatives within the resources available. Future planning prevents reliving the past. The planning ends with a *written* commitment, an action plan, with milestones and expected measurements of success.

As the plan is put into effect, constant evaluation is required to adjust to unforeseen challenges. In fact, in human healthcare only 20 percent of the changes have survived without major modification. But fear not, because another 30 percent survive with in process enhancements, caused by recurring evaluation techniques. As the process evolves and the project nears completion, study the outcomes. Evaluate the results for client benefit, staff benefit, and cost benefit. Although all three benefit evaluations need not be positive, the overall weighting must be positive (e.g., callbacks require initial training and extra time, but the staff is available anyway, and the clients appreciate the extra effort and tell their neighbors).

With habits, as with frozen clay and art sculptures, we must defrost, reshape, then refreeze to ensure that the new vision survives. This standardization is simply a recognition that the effort is worthwhile, so that others will realize the new system is the only one that will be used in the future. As with all things, today's innovation becomes tomorrow's mediocrity, so always be willing to change and make improvements continually, even if the system has been already addressed and revamped.

For instance, specialty practices seem to proliferate forms even faster than general veterinary practices. There is nothing wrong with the receptionist team being unilaterally accountable for the elimination of two forms in a quarter (consolidation of two into one is an elimination of one form). They know which ones are redundant for the clients (referring veterinarians or animal owners). The following quarter the technicians might attempt the same effort, eliminating two forms. If this secondary effort is successful, the receptionist team may try it again, or in a rare case, the doctors themselves might assess their own use of forms and eliminate two.

Quality Transformation—One Step at a Time

Unlike most programs, continuous quality improvement (CQI) is a perpetual process: one step at a time around the planning cycle of change. There may be a single starting point, but once begun, it should never end. In the process, please remember the story of the backpacking veterinarian who discovered it was not the height of the mountain that stopped the progress, but the grain of sand in the shoe.

Empower the team to remove the grains of sand whenever they find an irritation. Don't ask the staff to continue with an irritation; it only slows the eventual progress. In some cases the smallest irritant stops progress, and the status quo becomes the new practice plateau. To empower the staff is to let go of the process. The uncommon leader cares little for how the process occurs so long as the team follows acceptable practice quality standards and reaches the end point in a timely and appropriate manner. This is the leader who has excelled in defining end point expectations while making team members feel accountable for planning their own performance standards. This is the practice leader who can go home at nights without other people's problems on his or her mind. A true CQI practice encourages people to solve their own problems in a timely and caring manner. The leader recognizes the individual and the team and celebrates the effort, whether fully successful or not.

The uncommon leader understands that behavior rewarded is behavior repeated and takes action to stop negative reinforcement. Why have a sick-day program when a personal-day program can combine sick and vacation days together? *Sick days* reward sickness and absenteeism. Why give raises for tenure when performance can be tracked, like number of clients brought back to the practice by recall? Why bonus on gross income changes when, with proper budgeting, you can share savings or excess earnings with the team?

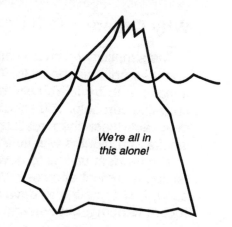

We're all in this alone!

Progress will come, one step at a time. The apple is eaten one bite at a time, but a single worm will stop the progress. The mountain is climbed one step at a time, but the grain of sand will stop the ascent. The continuous quality improvement process is one small project after another but can be halted by a leader who does not trust the team. Take your first step and celebrate with your team. Let them take their first step, then celebrate their effort. Soon your celebrations will be centered on change rather than on status quo, the mountain of problems will lie at your feet, and you will be soaring with the eagles.

CQI Checklists

Total quality management or continuous quality improvement takes time and an uncommon leadership. Between first hearing about it and doing something, there is often too long a period to keep enthusiasm high, so alternatives are needed. A personal-quality checklist often is a great tool to start the process and keep staff members involved while the leadership focuses on goals and objectives.

There are two broad types of job performance enhancements that the checklist system can help monitor: waste reducers or time savers (such as being on time for activities) and value-added activities (such as calling updates to clients). The first type helps staff members develop a personal understanding of quality in terms of their immediate work environment. This is valuable in its own right and leads to more effective team participation. But the checklist system is more than a training device. It can bring immediate and substantial improvements in personal job performance and satisfaction. However, improving job performance can't be the sole basis for judging the effectiveness of the CQI process. In fact, some have just recently realized it is a great suggestion program, as the organization culture becomes one of change rather than of status quo.

Why Create a CQI Checklist?

The simplicity of the personal CQI checklist often engenders skepticism about its potential benefits. The only way to convince yourself of its usefulness is to try it. You will be surprised how much and how quickly the checklist can help. You should first notice an improved ability to cope with daily activities, then realize the improvements can be maintained for weeks and months with little or no subsequent effort.

The hardest task is to develop a meaningful checklist. Actual data collection is almost effortless. You make a check mark when a defect is noticed. It is tempting to develop more elaborate systems that entail more record keeping, but beware. Such elaborate systems add little value and tend to collapse under the data-keeping burden. This seems to be the common thread of failure with many of the prepackaged time management systems. To develop the checklist around what you personally can control or change is critical. It requires insight into the job functions, and knowledge of the CQI principles.

How to Create the Checklist

Look at the incoming tasks first, those that come from others but are yours to resolve. Most can be done quickly but often are delayed due to poor work habits. The missing medical record is something we all have searched for just to find a two-minute entry holding up the filing. Concurrently, we have learned that working harder or faster is not the solution to the missing medical records. The best route to improvement is to eliminate the wasted effort in all its forms.

The personal CQI checklist starts with careful observation and reflection for about two or three weeks. Assemble the categories, borrow some from others if necessary, and tailor the words to your own environment. Study Table 4.1 and note that the defects are counted daily to track personal improvement.

If personal-quality checklists are used while the staff are trained on the principles of CQI, each staff member will gain personal experience with and belief in the process. The data could also be used for simple time-series analysis of trends associated with day-of-the-week effects or shift staffing habits. The weekly data charts can be amassed for monthly trends or long-term monitoring of lateral or vertical relationships.

The simple act of establishing the checklist will cause you to correct some habits immediately (Hawthorne Effect). Psychological research at the Hawthorne Supply Depot showed that if people thought they were being watched or studied, whether they were or not, their performance improved. Some categories will self-correct, and others will need specific attention to resolve. Don't be surprised if the majority of the categories self-correct almost immediately.

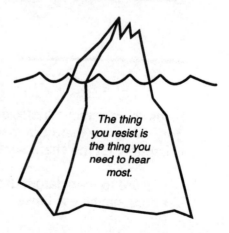

The thing
you resist is
the thing you
need to hear
most.

The checklist adds a calming effect, as, by definition, everything can't be done at once. The temptation to try is mediated by the check marks indicating effort in the daily schedule. The chaos becomes controlled. Gains will not be measured solely in defect reduction. The checklist permits people to watch themselves as they do things and

Table 4.1. The Personal CQI Checklist

| Rebecca the Receptionist's Personal CQI Checklist | | | | | | Week of _____ | | |
DEFECT CATEGORY	MON	TUE	WED	THU	FRI	SAT	SUN	TOTAL
Late* for Meeting, Appt., or Duty Shift								
Search* for Something Lost, Misplaced								
Delayed* Return of Telephone Call or Callback								
Put a Small Task on Hold*								
Failure to Discard* Incoming Junk on Front Counter								
Miss a Chance* to Clean the Office or Waiting Area								
Unnecessary Inspection*								

Definitions:
* Late = even by one minute
* Search = more than momentary confusion, includes forgetting a task
* Delay = failure to act at first opportunity
* Put on Hold = quick action, like file a folder, is put on a stack
* Discard = failure to react to clutter, junk is not friendly
* Miss a Chance = any delay in cleaning, dusting, or pickup
* Inspection = checking something already done but didn't pay attention first time

helps them remove inefficiencies not directly covered in a specific category. Because there are many categories other than what I have already illustrated, let me share some:

- failure to meet target dates
- personal fitness lapses

- failure to listen closely
- procrastination
- failure to seek self-improvement weekly
- making typos, misdialing or other "too fast" errors
- failure to recover promptly from interruptions

These concepts are not new. Ben Franklin noted in his autobiography that there were 13 categories to pursue in the search for improved character and behavior:

- temperance
- silence
- order
- resolution
- frugality
- industry
- sincerity
- justice
- moderation
- cleanliness
- tranquility
- chastity
- humility

Ben also noted that pride often gets in the way of improvement of character and behavior and wrote, "In reality, there is, perhaps, not one of our natural passions so hard to subdue as pride . . . even if I could conceive that I had completely overcome it, I should probably be proud of my humility."

Taking a cue from Franklin, I offer here nine more negative character and behavior categories to consider avoiding for your checklist:

- unkind humor
- defeatism
- worry
- griping
- flustering
- sarcasm
- unpleasantness

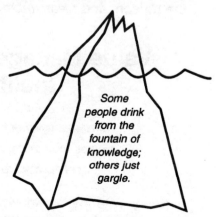

Some people drink from the fountain of knowledge; others just gargle.

• disagreeable tone of voice
• dishonesty

You might think a mere checklist could not change behavior or character, but if the checklist is firmly embedded in your consciousness, the possibility of a defect is a strong deterrent to undesirable behavior. Think of it. If you start to feel sorry for yourself, you are giving in to defeatism, and the average person will reject the feeling, start another project, or pursue a new goal rather than give him- or herself a check mark.

How Long Until Perfection?

How far should you go to reduce personal defects? One school of thought says you should never stop. Perfection is the goal; reducing defects annually is the method. But if you believe in CQI, the checklist will change, priorities will lead to newly added items, perhaps replacing distracting habits that have been corrected. Continuous quality improvement will not allow the checklist to be a static set of categories. Some people even have a "retired category" checklist, a list of old habits on a secondary checklist, just in case reversion may attack later.

The initial calming effects and the ongoing improvement provides encouragement to continue, but the leadership must support the process. The operational definitions of each category must be established before the process starts, and that may take some brainstorming with the boss to ensure the environment will support the effort. Another problem is an imbalance between time wasters and value-added activities. Time must be made available before new ideas can be added, and a good leader will help maintain awareness of the need for the balance. A caring leader will help ensure that the goals are *R*ealistic for the environment, *A*ttainable for the person, and *M*easurable (RAM the CQI process).

Value Management with Continuous Quality Improvement

Value management is a step-by-step creative process that revolves around the word "function." It helps the staff identify better ways to effect necessary critical change.

Every veterinarian knows a three-legged milking stool is far steadier than a one-, two- or four-legged version when trying to get the job done.

Why then, do most practice veterinarians ignore the other two support legs when addressing improvements needed within a practice? We realize that without clients, we don't have a practice, so they are one leg, but they are seldom used in managing change. How often does your practice team forget that clients are a critical leg of a practice support system? The veterinarian is always one leg of the support system, usually by the owner's definition—right or wrong! The paraprofessional staff forms the third leg of any support system, because without them, the job seldom gets done. Inversely, the paraprofessional staff are frequently ignored in the problem-solving process.

History Does Repeat Itself

At the turn of the century, Lister and Company was Britain's leading silk supplier with incredible profits; they set the standard for corporations. In 1912 a company chemist, Samuel Courtauld, suggested to management that a synthetic silk was possible. The corporate leaders tore Courtauld's idea to shreds, insisting the public would never accept the inferior product. Sam listened to their counsel, quit Lister and Company, and proceeded to take his new synthetic silk, called rayon, to the public; his multimillion dollar success story was the result.

Once there was a guy who tried to peddle a great chicken recipe and no one would buy it, so he built a little store and sold chicken cooked with his recipe; the Kentucky Fried Chicken success story is history.

A quiet 3M chemist couldn't get the glue to dry, so he reapplied it to only specific parts of the paper, and we have had "sticky notes" ever since.

Similar veterinary medical examples abound:

- A frustrated practitioner didn't fire two employees because he thought he was at fault. After deliberation with a consultant, and establishing that his values were critical to success, he let them go, the practice energy increased, and he went from one stagnant practice to six thriving practices in two years.

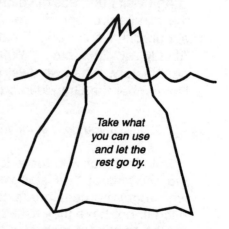

Take what you can use and let the rest go by.

- After over two years of no practice growth, low liquidity, and poor practice harmony, a practitioner decided to ask a consultant for help. In trying new methods to get clients through the door, the team tripled the number of new clients and increased harmony; he took a four-week vacation and the practice continued to improve. When he returned, he decided the success of the practice was not worth the changes he had to make in his personal style, and he reverted, losing most of his staff in the process. My consulting team did disengage from this practice because our trust in his values had also been lost.

■ The single owner of a mixed practice (dairy heavy) wanted the associate to buy in, but the liquidity for two owners didn't exist. A competitor with five practitioners moved in across the street; panic set in. The two called in a consultant who found that the practice was stagnant. The competition in large animals was significant. In the 30-mile radius around the practice, there was only one small-animal practitioner, with an average to marginal practice approach to companion animal care. The new associate had a small-animal interest, but they had never considered this a viable option. An assessment of the owner's and associate's practice values uncovered a genuine pride in their small-animal care, and this interest allowed them to research and embrace the tactics necessary to improve the liquidity to allow the buy-in to occur from the new revenues.

■ After three years of no fiscal growth, a veterinarian and his wife sought assistance; they wanted a quick fix. The wife knew she had to do the management for her husband; he had a learning disability. The wife's ability to keep everything in control was exacting and total. The practice ceased to change and adapt to the environment. The husband continued to practice longer and harder but could not change the trends. His consultant encouraged him to clarify his expectations and values, and this helped him increase the annual value of his average practice client by 40 percent.

As I visit hundreds of veterinary practices, I find it interesting to observe the mind-set of specific key leaders within the practice. The trite phases abound: "It won't work," "That's not our style," "It's too late," "We can't ...," "If only ...," "Yes, but ..." When we look only backward in time, we will repeat history. When we dwell on what could have been, we get no further. Remember the Granddad quote from Chapter 1?

If you don't stand for something, you will fall for anything.

Veterinarians who make too many management decisions aren't using the services of their staff very well. There are even a few veterinarians who *require* a certain outpatient appointment log format but have never used it, nor have they asked the front team to improve it. The same goes for the treatment-room day sheet; technicians are seldom, if ever, asked to improve it! Anyone can make decisions. Just ask the kennel supervisor if you should buy a new computer, and you'll probably get an answer; but this is not a decision, it is a guess. Most good decisions are self-evident based on the research and background knowledge of the hospital staff.

Just to ensure you do not think veterinary medicine is alone in its accumulation of control freaks, author Al Kelly, in the text *How to Make Your Life Easier at Work*, looked at the frequency with which managers said no to requests and ideas submitted to them, and categorized the managers according to their frequency of *no* answers:

20 percent *no* replies—Either you have a selection of idiots reporting to you, or you are one yourself and don't know what's going on.

5 percent *no* replies—You are asserting the veto to prove your presence.

1 percent *no* replies —This is tolerable in a rapidly changing environment and if the "no" means there is a need for additions or alterations before approval.

0.1 percent *no* replies—This is about normal.

0.0 percent *no* replies—You are a rubber stamp (and in this context, that's good).

Another common alternative to the fast-draw "no" in a practice is the management excuse based on superior experience. Sometimes, the staff sees it as paralysis by analysis. We call these types of attitudes The Dirty Dozen of stagnation. (These are not to be confused with The Dirty Dozen Questions and associated tables in Chapter 3.)

Disqualifying: "That couldn't be implemented here."

Editing: "That is a great idea but won't work in this area."

All-or-nothing thinking: "If we can't do it 100 percent, we won't try it."

Uncritical acceptance of critics: "They have said it isn't smart."

Perfectionism: "I need more information on how to ensure success."

Fortune-telling: "I'll never get my clients to accept that."

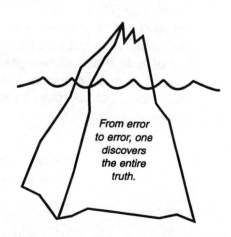

From error to error, one discovers the entire truth.

Overgeneralization: "If we did that, we wouldn't have time to breathe."

Emotional reasoning: "I know we'd never be happy doing it that way."

Labeling: "That is unethical advertising."

Personalization: "If I did that my colleagues would ..."

Minimizing: "We could try it, but it wouldn't make a great difference."

Complacency: "I am happy with what I've done to get here, so we don't need to change."

Eliminate Excuses

Many things get in the way of doing a task as it ought to be done: work overload, understaffing, too many bosses, short on resources, too many rules, not enough experience, improper training, ineffective leadership, and so on. Staff members also may come to the practice handicapped with personal problems or a poor attitude. It is impossible to eliminate all the factors that may make it difficult for a staff member to do a superior job. But it is possible to help that person become more productive in spite of those factors.

Practices that blame external circumstances, such as staff problems or slowed growth, are not looking for solutions. In the analysis phase, remember: only 20 percent of the facts will impact on 80 percent of the outcome. So try it; then be ready to adjust for new discoveries. Those who want all the facts or never to make a mistake are setting themselves up for failure. As they say in the dairy industry, "Don't cry over spilt milk; just find another cow to milk."

Problems prevent good performance only when they become excuses for not trying to improve. Use the phrase "given that..." when you address the next set of excuses you hear. "Given that" statements acknowledge real handicaps, yet insist the staff member find a way to be more productive despite those challenges; they are a powerful way to remove the excuse so that a productive discussion about how to improve performance can occur. Let us repeat the quote from Thomas Jefferson, which appeared in Chapter 1:

> *In matters of style, swim with the current;*
> *in matters of principle, stand like a rock.*

A common example is the veterinarian who says, "The clients can't afford that level of care; we offer Cadillac care to a Yugo population." Instead, think in these terms: "I know it would be easier if every client loved his or her pet like a family member and had the money to keep it in perfect health, but since that's not the case, what can be done to improve the standard of preventive and forensic medicine offerings to a level that helps the pet and still considers the economic plight of the clients?"

"Given that" statements eliminate long and unproductive discussions about how bad things are or about whether a staff member is justified in being frustrated. They also shift the responsibility back to the staff member to improve performance despite handicaps.

Bottom Line

In the case of excuses, one thing remains constant. The target must be well defined by the leader of the practice. No member of the staff can be expected to pursue practice goals if they are kept a secret, remain ill defined, or are not put in measurable terms. If the ownership decides to target a certain level of healthcare as the standard, then that is the measurement that must be used. Excuses for falling short of that goal need to be eliminated.

A set of practice values is a simple set of beliefs—nothing more, but nothing less. They start with the visionary but must be embraced by all the team. They are a constant yardstick used to measure the quality of care to clients, patients, and each other. If someone follows the values, what they do cannot be wrong, even if it does not work. In the past we have shared three sets of value crutches:

Q = quality	P = patient	C = client
U = understanding	R = respect	A = action
E = excellence	I = innovation	R = respect
S = service	D = dedication	E = excellence
T = teamwork	E = excellence	

It doesn't matter what you use (McDonald's uses Q-V-S-C, as in quality-value-service-cleanliness), as long as you *never* allow a violation to pass without comment. These are the elements of consistency that support the practice philosophy (mission statement), and all staff members

If you love what you do, you will never work another day in your life!

need to depend upon the support of the leadership when they use a value in making a practice decision.

We have discussed methods to eliminate the mistaken thought processes that become detrimental habits, but some staff members will not respond to coaching or to "given that" acknowledgments. An astute manager must realize that they are probably in the wrong practice, and maybe even in the wrong profession. A good leader will help those staff members who want assistance to learn how to reach the practice target (goals and objectives). A good leader will also eliminate those who won't accept the practice target as appropriate to their values. The values of the leadership make the practice philosophy come alive and allow the staff unilaterally to select new methods effecting continuous quality improvement within their scope of accountability, responsibility, and daily operations. Remember Grandma:

If you were to sell your character,
would you get full retail,
or
would it go for a bargain-basement
price with discount coupons?

■ ■ ■ Review ■ ■ ■

In this chapter we've covered the information that supports the idea of "training to trust" before you delegate responsibilities to your staff. This nurturing of your leadership competencies has been described using the Competencies Iceberg. We've also given you examples of how a leader nurtures through a core set of competencies, a chart of the levels of leadership, and the CQI checklist. With this information you can now tie up the process of basic leadership and team-building principles presented in the previous three lessons.

As you work with your own staff to incorporate these principles, always keep in mind that teams are dynamic, not static. Your position as team leader gives you many opportunities to defy traditional attitudes of office management and create an environment that brings efficiency to the practice and quality service to the clients and patients.

1. Continuous quality improvement is not a program; it is a commitment to your team, your clients, and yourself to make change the norm.

2. The *L* in "quality" stands for leadership because leaders must be committed to nurturing others.

3. Clients can judge pride, not quality; they perceive staff pride as verification of quality in a practice.

4. Six leadership factors
   a. Preach and lead with a vision.
   b. Set the example and practice what you preach.
   c. Make people accountable.
   d. Empower your staff.
   e. Take risks!
   f. Go for the long haul, not the quick fix.

5. Ten pillars of CQI
   a. Trust in values
   b. Commitment
   c. Accountability
   d. Recognition
   e. Training
   f. Communication
   g. Reminders
   h. Expectations
   i. Evaluation
   j. Problem solving

6. Habits are icebergs waiting to be thawed, changed, and reshaped.

7. CQI Planning Process Preparation has three steps:
   a. Take the TPR out of your practice.
   b. Characterize your staff.
   c. Identify components of a best-fit strategy.

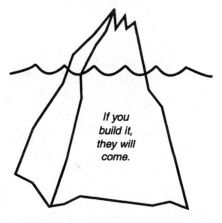

If you build it, they will come.

Dare to Ask for Feedback

TEAM READINESS

(For clarity, use different-colored paper for each form.)

1. The Staff Opinion Survey, with Philosophy of Practice, the Leadership Feasibility Audit, and the Soft Skills Inventory should be distributed first and filled out anonymously. Then they are collected and held for the leadership team's review. This gives you the baseline needed, before starting the four-stage Team Readiness Assessment.

2. The Stage 1 Team Readiness Assessment should be the agenda handout before the first CQI meeting you hold, and collected after that meeting in exchange for the Stage 2 Team Readiness Assessment.

3. At the staff meeting a month later, the Stage 2 Team Readiness Assessment should be collected before the meeting. If there isn't a meeting, this collection still becomes a practice leadership responsibility for the end of the first month. Regardless, the Stage 3 Team Readiness Assessment needs to be distributed after Stage 2 is collected, to be completed and returned before the next staff meeting in another month.

4. Within the first quarter, the practice leader will hold a team core values/vision meeting (use the Effective Team Meetings for planning) and will use the Team Meeting Assessment form to evaluate it before the team members depart. The leader will collect Stage 3 and then distribute the Stage 4 Team Readiness Assessment as a form exchange at the end of the meeting. Forms need to be collected anonymously.

5. The next team meeting will be facilitated by a staff member. Ensure that the person facilitating the meeting has the Effective Team Meetings I and II to plan, and ensure that he or she uses it. The main meeting agenda item will be the frequency and format of team meetings. Allow the staff facilitator to first distribute the Decision Time—Staff Buy-in Effective Team Meeting II chart and review with the team the previously completed Team Meeting Assessment results. Then the facilitator will handle the agenda item (frequency and format) by leading a team discussion about problem solving at team meetings—what kind, how to offer ideas, how to respect others, and how to reach a practice-benefit decision. The Consensus Assessment form will be used to evaluate the outcome of that discussion and the team meeting chart Assertive–Cooperative, the Effective Team Meeting III summary, will be distributed to each person, as one among the group will be the next facilitator to volunteer.

6. The Performance Appraisal in a CQI-Based Team introduces a new look at the old score card appraisals. This complex overview is simplified and explained in more detail in Volume 2 of this leadership series.

STAFF OPINION SURVEY

Instructions: Please read each statement carefully. Then circle the response that best expresses your feelings about the statement.

	Strongly Agree	Agree Somewhat /Usually	Neither Agree nor Disagree	Disagree Somewhat /Usually	Strongly Disagree
1. I have the information I need to do my job properly.	5	4	3	2	1
2. I know my supervisor's expectations of my work.	5	4	3	2	1
3. My personal work effort contributes to this practice's success.	5	4	3	2	1
4. There are reasonable opportunities to improve my personal performance in this practice.	5	4	3	2	1
5. Salary increases here are based on merit and job-oriented qualifications.	5	4	3	2	1
6. Staff members who perform well are given more responsibility and recognition.	5	4	3	2	1
7. I understand the work rules and policies of this practice.	5	4	3	2	1
8. Our philosophy of practice applies to all members of the staff and veterinarians equally.	5	4	3	2	1
9. Concerned patient care is conveyed to our clients at every opportunity.	5	4	3	2	1
10. This is a safe place to work.	5	4	3	2	1
11. I have a clear understanding of the benefit plan here.	5	4	3	2	1
12. There are no favorites or discrimination in this practice.	5	4	3	2	1

132

	Strongly Agree	Agree Somewhat /Usually	Neither Agree nor Disagree	Disagree Somewhat /Usually	Strongly Disagree
13. Generally, the doctors set a good example and practice tone.	5	4	3	2	1
14. The middle-management decisions of this practice usually make sense to me.	5	4	3	2	1
15. The management-staff relationship here is good.	5	4	3	2	1
16. I feel free to discuss my problems with the doctor.	5	4	3	2	1
17. The veterinarian's recognition comes quickly when I do a good job.	5	4	3	2	1
18. They praise us in public and correct in private in this practice.	5	4	3	2	1
19. My middle manager knows his/her job very well.	5	4	3	2	1
20. I get plenty of help improving my performance.	5	4	3	2	1
21. I understand the practice's goals and objectives.	5	4	3	2	1
22. The goals and objectives of my job are in tune with the practice's goals and objectives.	5	4	3	2	1
23. Communication between the staff members is good.	5	4	3	2	1
24. Client communications are a high-interest concern of this practice.	5	4	3	2	1
25. I believe the results of this survey will be used constructively by this practice.	5	4	3	2	1

Please write any comments you may have on the back. All responses will be kept strictly confidential and will not be quoted verbatim.

PHILOSOPHY OF PRACTICE

JOB TITLE_____

To help identify your practice philosophy and mission statement, please answer the following questions with a few descriptive, informative sentences. Individuals' names should not be used. To be completed by each staff member.

A. Please list the three highest-priority goals for this practice for the next year (short-term goals).

    1._____

    _____

    2._____

    _____

    3._____

    _____

B. What is your most significant contribution to the practice in each of the above-mentioned areas?

    _____

    _____

    _____

    _____

    _____

    _____

C. Please list the three highest-priority goals for this practice for the next three years (long-term goals).

    1._____

    _____

    2._____

    _____

    3._____

    _____

D. What is your most significant contribution to the practice in each of the above-mentioned areas?

    _____

    _____

    _____

    _____

    _____

    _____

LEADERSHIP FEASIBILITY AUDIT

(Leaders only)

Circle one response number for each statement as it applies to this inventory.

SA (4) = Strongly agree - You strongly agree with the statement.
A   (3) = Agree - You agree more than you disagree with the statement.
D   (2) = Disagree - You disagree more than you agree with the statement.
SD (1) = Strongly disagree - You strongly disagree with the statement.
NA (0) = Not applicable - The statement does not apply.

	SA	A	D	SD	NA
1. Our work tasks are compatible with a team-oriented system.	4	3	2	1	0
2. Our staff members are willing to participate and take risks.	4	3	2	1	0
3. Our staff members are skilled enough to participate technically, interpersonally, and administratively.	4	3	2	1	0
4. Our philosophy will allow us to renegotiate job classifications and work rules.	4	3	2	1	0
5. Our supervisors display good interpersonal and listening skills and can be supportive.	4	3	2	1	0
6. Our practice has a history of following through on changes.	4	3	2	1	0
7. Our practice will view this consultation as a cultural shift rather than just as a new program.	4	3	2	1	0
8. Our culture and policies could be converted to a more integrated team system (empowerment, recognition, communication, and change).	4	3	2	1	0
9. Our market can support additional veterinary services.	4	3	2	1	0
10. We are ready and willing to face the challenges of self-directed teams, realizing that it is a lengthy, challenging process.	4	3	2	1	0

SOFT SKILLS INVENTORY

(Everyone)

I am a ___ doctor ___ receptionist ___ technician ___ assistant

Rate the following inventory for yourself as well as for your team in the area of soft skills (people skills), with 1 being least skilled and 5 being most skilled. Use a circle to identify yourself and a square to identify your team.

○ Me   ❑ My Team

	Least				Most
Listening carefully to what others have to say	1	2	3	4	5
Seeking consensus rather than making unilateral decisions	1	2	3	4	5
Sharing information instead of hoarding it	1	2	3	4	5
Accepting individual differences	1	2	3	4	5
Resolving conflict cleanly	1	2	3	4	5
Controlling one's attitude (self-discipline)	1	2	3	4	5
Accepting change	1	2	3	4	5
Selling ideas	1	2	3	4	5
Facilitating (lead discussion by asking questions)	1	2	3	4	5
Coaching and encouraging	1	2	3	4	5
Leading productive meetings	1	2	3	4	5
Negotiating win/win	1	2	3	4	5
Using eye contact / smiles / nods	1	2	3	4	5
Being attentive to personal grooming	1	2	3	4	5
Crediting the team rather than seeking personal glory	1	2	3	4	5
Remaining open to team suggestions	1	2	3	4	5
Maintaining overall interpersonal skills (people skills)	1	2	3	4	5

TEAM READINESS ASSESSMENT: STAGE 1

(Distribute after Soft Skills collected.)

ANONYMOUS

Place an X on the line at the point that best indicates your level of agreement with the statement.

	POOR	NEUTRAL	GREAT
1. I understand what self-directed continuous quality improvement (CQI) is.	|———|———|———|
2. I believe CQI teams will work well here.	|———|———|———|
3. I will fully support the team approach.	|———|———|———|
4. I trust team members will appropriately use team resources.	|———|———|———|
5. I think teams will benefit me personally.	|———|———|———|
6. I believe that most people here can work well in self-directed work teams.	|———|———|———|
7. I understand how teams are led, facilitated, and coached.	|———|———|———|
8. I agree with the daily, weekly, monthly time line for self-directed CQI teams.	|———|———|———|
9. I understand and agree with the team member selection criteria.	|———|———|———|

Action Items to Catalyze Progression to Stage 2:

_____

_____

_____

_____

_____

TEAM READINESS ASSESSMENT: STAGE 2

ANONYMOUS

Place an X on the line at the point that best indicates your level of agreement with the statement.

	POOR	NEUTRAL	GREAT

1. I understand the objectives and goals of this team.

2. I consider the objectives and goals of this team to be reasonable.

3. I believe in the vision, mission, and values of this organization.

4. I know what is expected of me personally in this team approach.

5. I know which functions (once performed by the supervisors and managers) will eventually be shifted to the team.

6. I will participate in and use scheduled training.

7. I agree that we can make teams succeed without sacrificing quality or customer service.

8. I believe that our leaders can truly coach and encourage us to succeed.

9. The selection of the team leader is clear and appropriate.

10. I consider others on the team to be competent and trustworthy.

Action Items to Catalyze Progression to Stage 3:

_____

_____

_____

TEAM READINESS ASSESSMENT: STAGE 3

ANONYMOUS

Place an X on the line at the point that best indicates your level of agreement with the statement.

	POOR	NEUTRAL	GREAT

1. We know when to make our own decisions and when to consult others.

2. We keep the mentor updated frequently.

3. We conduct meaningful, effective meetings.

4. We each know what is expected of us.

5. We have visited other team-based organizations.

6. We have a clear team mission statement.

7. We feel supported by our mentor and management leadership.

8. We make suggestions that are listened to and implemented.

9. We are kept informed and are connected to other parts of the organization.

10. We are recognized and encouraged for our accomplishments.

Action Items to Catalyze Progression to Stage 4:

_____

_____

_____

_____

TEAM READINESS ASSESSMENT: STAGE 4

ANONYMOUS

Place an X on the line at the point that best indicates your level of agreement with the statement.

| | POOR | NEUTRAL | GREAT |

1. We will rotate job responsibilities and assignments throughout the team as needed.

    ├──────────┼──────────┤

2. We will be able to reach consensus on most issues.

    ├──────────┼──────────┤

3. We freely support other staff members and doctors.

    ├──────────┼──────────┤

4. We are accepted and supported by others on our team.

    ├──────────┼──────────┤

5. We will rotate team leaders, mentors, and meeting facilitators appropriately.

    ├──────────┼──────────┤

6. We will regularly exceed service expectations and quality schedules.

    ├──────────┼──────────┤

7. We are measured and rewarded on teamwork, not only on individual performance.

    ├──────────┼──────────┤

8. We are open to new team members and share our members with other teams as required.

    ├──────────┼──────────┤

9. We celebrate ourselves and our accomplishments regularly.

    ├──────────┼──────────┤

10. We continuously learn and apply ways to improve everything.

    ├──────────┼──────────┤

Action Items to Catalyze Further Progression:

_____

_____

_____

Team Multivoting

1. *Select a facilitator and recorder.*
2. *Brainstorm a list of nine specific events, trends, issues, or recurring problems affecting your workplace or practice.*
3. *Vote the list down to three items; each team member votes for his or her top three items.*
4. *The three items with the most votes are selected.*
5. *Prioritize the list of three items from 3 to 1 (1 being most important).*
6. *Generate a potential solution or opportunity for item number one.*
7. *Specify several action steps or tactics—things to do within 90 days—for this potential solution or opportunity.*

Events or problems	Each team member votes for three events						Total votes
	#1*	#2	#3	#4	#5	#6	
1.							
2.							
3.							
4.							
5.							
6.							
7.							
8.							
9.							

*Team member #1, etc.

Possible solution: _____

Action steps to reach solution:

_____

_____

NOTE: Success measurements need to be agreed upon (known) *before* starting.

_____

_____

EFFECTIVE TEAM MEETINGS: 2

(Time required to arrive at a decision)

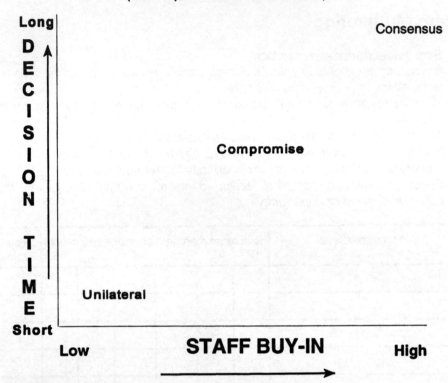

Facilitators

1. Explain task
2. Clarify ground rules
   (no one 2x until all 1x)
3. Lead an icebreaker
4. Include all
5. Help group deal with dominators

6. Keep pace
7. Refocus
8. Help group reward
9. Catalyze follow-up assignments
10. Ensure all understand assignments
11. Encourage the caring heart

Norms for team meetings

1. Establish team board room
2. Start and end on time
3. Rotate facilitator
4. Arrange for personal needs
5. Encourage disagreements
6. Discourage parking lot agendas

7. Deal directly with problem
   performance
8. Allow probing questions
9. Develop an action plan
10. Follow up on the action plan
11. Reduce doctor input

The five functional roles in a team meeting

1. Facilitator—neutral
2. Timekeeper—functionally
   neutral

3. Recorder—functionally neutral
4. Owner(s)—not neutral
5. Resources—not neutral

TEAM MEETING ASSESSMENT

ANONYMOUS

- *Copy and disseminate this assessment to team members when necessary.*
- *Collect and summarize their anonymous responses.*
- *Brainstorm Action Items to improve weak areas.*
- *Brainstorm Action Items to celebrate strong areas.*

	EXCELLENT	GOOD	FAIR	POOR	
1. Purpose of Meetings					
Clear	❏	❏	❏	❏	Not defined
2. Participation in Meetings					
Shared by all	❏	❏	❏	❏	Dominated by a few
3. Preparedness for Meetings					
Ready to interact	❏	❏	❏	❏	Never ready
4. Agenda					
Prepublished and on time	❏	❏	❏	❏	Nonexistent or late
5. Action Plan					
Updated and disseminated	❏	❏	❏	❏	Nonexistent or late
6. Time					
Allocated wisely	❏	❏	❏	❏	Too haphazardly allocated
7. Creativity					
Open and fresh	❏	❏	❏	❏	Boring/stuck
8. Consensus					
Everyone supports decisions	❏	❏	❏	❏	Unilateral/parking lot agendas
9. Facilitators					
Rotate enough	❏	❏	❏	❏	Stuck with same
Remain neutral	❏	❏	❏	❏	Lose objectivity
Inspire new insights	❏	❏	❏	❏	Follow old pattern
Appoint timekeeper and recorder	❏	❏	❏	❏	Do it all themselves
Are trained	❏	❏	❏	❏	Are not skilled
10. The Coach					
Always present	❏	❏	❏	❏	Never see him or her
Too involved	❏	❏	❏	❏	Too detached
Encourages us	❏	❏	❏	❏	Demotivates us
Helps us	❏	❏	❏	❏	Abandons us

EFFECTIVE TEAM MEETINGS: 3
(Types of decision making)

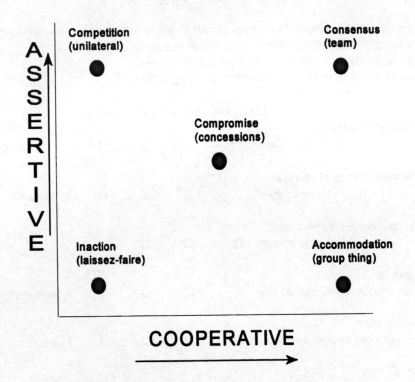

Consensus

1. We all will support 100 percent.
2. We all must agree at least 75 percent.
3. Anyone can block a team vote by offering a reasonable alternative.
4. Members who habitually block without alternatives or demonstrate demoralizing behavior can be voted off the team.
5. There will be no parking lot agendas.

CONSENSUS ASSESSMENT
Team exercise (role clarification)

INSTRUCTIONS: *Each member of the team should fill out this assessment after a consensus has been reached. Calculate your score, add to the total score of the other team members, then divide that number by the number of people on your team.*

		1	2	3	
Participation	one-sided	❑	❑	❑	equal
Ideas generated	few	❑	❑	❑	many
Trust and respect expressed	minimal	❑	❑	❑	frequent
Decision based on blend of ideas	no	❑	❑	❑	yes
Support of team decision	low	❑	❑	❑	high

My score: _____

Total team score: _____

Average score: _____
(Total score divided by the number of team members)

How well did your team create a consensus? An average score in the range of 12 to 15 (assuming a team of five members*) would indicate a good consensus process, whereas a range of 9 to 11 would indicate you need to look at specific areas for improvement (e.g., participation) and practice these.

How could the team have improved the consensus process?

*If your team has more members, adjust these score ranges by multiplying the number of members by 5, then dividing that total into thirds.

PERFORMANCE APPRAISAL IN A CQI-BASED TEAM

*The coach appraises the team. The **mature** team appraises its members.*

	Informal	Formal
☐ **Who**	Everyone related to team.	Two reviewers: one selected by person being reviewed, one elected by team.
☐ **When**	Once per month at "housekeeping meeting."	Once per quarter for detailed plan. Once per year for annual plan.
☐ **How**	Team leader asks: • "What have we heard are our strengths?" • "What have we heard are our areas for improvement?" Individual plans include:	Quarterly team plan is revised or generated with the mentor. Annual individual plans are generated by partitioning the team plan.

• Objectives (what is expected)
• Standards (how work is to be done in qualitative teams)

• Training to be completed
• Areas for improvement

Monthly "projections" are conducted at "housekeeping meetings" so there are no surprises.

Annually, reviewers survey team members and all associated with team to evaluate perspectives of team members' performance.

Team member completes evaluation of his or her performance.

Evaluations are compared, settlement is reached between reviewers and individual team members.

The team members' share of team compensation may be influenced by this appraisal.

☐ **What**

Technical
• Strengths
• Areas for improvements

Administrative
• Strengths
• Areas for improvement

Interpersonal
• Strengths
• Areas for improvements

Work habits
• Strengths
• Areas for improvement

This Appendix contains samples of handouts that can be used with your staff for each leadership skill mentioned in Chapter 2. When possible, a single picture is used in lieu of a thousand words.

KNOWING AND USING THE RESOURCES OF THE GROUP

Resource material includes: reference books, continuing education, money, tools, time, calendars, local associations, clients, experiences, libraries, volunteers, staff, consultants, equipment, community leaders, knowledge, and other people, programs, or things that may assist in accomplishing the desired outcome.

All employees bring strengths with them. The leader searches for strengths and builds upon them. These strengths may be physical, social, or ethical; they may also be hobbies, experiences, skills, or other mental strengths. New perspectives, alternatives, and innovative ideas are resources to cherish and nurture. "Ethics in Action" means to cherish and nurture the other person as a valuable resource, and know that personal values are irreplaceable resources.

Effective recruitment of resources means to ask, not to tell. It means soliciting other opinions and avoiding the conclusion that staff members are wrong when they disagree. Programs built upon the resource strengths of the staff have a far greater success rate than systems given to the staff or programs designed to address a weakness within the group.

A leader who truly knows him- or herself seeks others who add to the capability resources of the group. New leaders are constantly under development as additional resources within the group. As a practice grows, the owner control of the early years must give way to team control, so leaders must be developed from within the staff. This is a never-ending quest for the caring leader of quality healthcare teams.

EFFECTIVE COMMUNICATION
Getting and Giving Information

Written, spoken, seen, heard, smelled, or whatever, information is conveyed in a continuous flow. Note taking helps retain ideas, and a picture (sketch) may be worth a thousand words—but to communicate, another person is required!

▼ VERBAL

● VOCAL

■ VISUAL

The key success ingredient to effective communication is believability. UCLA research has shown that silent messages confuse the information receiver, as the interpersonal message is most often

▼ 7 percent verbal

● 38 percent vocal

■ 55 percent visual

Stanford has demonstrated that the most successful communicators have three personal qualities that have positive effects on their careers:

• An outgoing, ascendant personality

• A desire to persuade, to talk, and to work with people

• A need for power

Your listeners won't care what you know (or say) until they know that you care. Never bluff a staff member; never lie to a client—it is okay to say "I don't know." Clients always have the right to say no, so always give them two "yes" alternatives, then be quiet and listen. Staff and clients know the truth when they hear it and deserve at least that much, at all times, in healthcare situations.

Stand tall; be proud of yourself and your practice. Be able to face the person in the mirror each morning with the same open pride. The difference between towering and cowering is totally a matter of inner posture. It's got nothing to do with height, it costs nothing, and it's more fun!

UNDERSTANDING THE CHARACTERISTICS AND NEEDS OF THE GROUP

Know yourself ... characteristics (the "what is") contain needs (the "something missing") ... leaders understand the difference and try to respond to both.

Leaders are sensitive to the needs of others by understanding the characteristics of each person, as well as of the group. The needs of the individual are often hidden behind the needs of the group. The CQI "teeter-totter" holds individual needs on one end and group needs on the other; understanding the balance is the first step in forming a group.

individual_____group

During the group-forming stage, a caring leader continually strives to rebalance the teeter-totter. Individual needs must be addressed by the group, just as group needs must be accepted by the individual. Leaders are constantly facilitating these discussions and changes.

The priorities for any caring group are determined by remaining aware of the characteristics and needs of the individual at the same time you remain aware of the characteristics and needs of the group.

Whereas characteristics seldom change quickly, needs are dynamic and continually change. The most effective leaders fulfill those unmet needs.

The balance between addressing individual needs and group needs is one of the hardest leadership tasks within new groups. Group priorities must address both sets of needs for the leader to be perceived as caring and believable.

REFLECTING

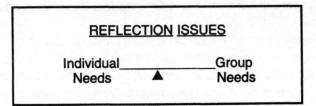

REFLECTION ISSUES

Individual_____Group
Needs   ▲   Needs

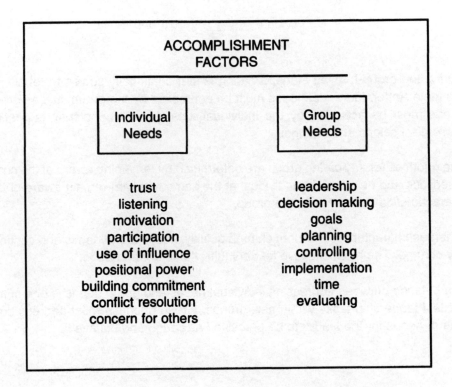

ACCOMPLISHMENT
FACTORS

Individual Needs	Group Needs
trust	leadership
listening	decision making
motivation	goals
participation	planning
use of influence	controlling
positional power	implementation
building commitment	time
conflict resolution	evaluating
concern for others	

Use empathy (feeling), caring (guiding), and open-ended questions.

Maintaining the balance between nurturing the individual and keeping the group together is the secret of effective leadership, especially with staff and young veterinarians.

REPRESENTING THE GROUP

Effective use of this leadership skill relies on the presence of the previous four skills. In representation, there is always resistance to overcome, and a good leader will know the characteristics and needs of those involved, seek resources, reflect on alternatives, develop new goals, and communicate believability and caring.

The toughest skill for the new practice leader is to wear the two hats of leadership:

1. Representing the peer group, their wants, needs, and desires, to the doctor(s), practice owner, other staff elements, practice manager, and outside world, and
2. Representing and selling the programs of the doctor(s), practice owner, other staff elements, practice manager, and outside world to other members of the staff (the peer group).

Although a consulting method of representation is preferred, this is not always possible, so being aware of the characteristics and needs of the group and of individual staff members helps a leader better represent the group. Knowing the available resources within the group also helps the leader make commitments when consulting is not possible.

Communicating positively is critical to selling new ideas and is a skill that requires practice and rehearsal. This means knowing what other people want and presenting the alternatives in terms that, from their point of view, are friendly.

The knowledge and use of this skill is an operational cornerstone when building the leaders and practices of tomorrow.

PLANNING

Done by the staff members, for their programs.

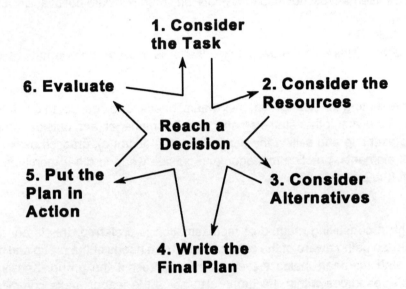

REMEMBER ALWAYS—THE ROOTS OF PLANNING INCLUDE:

**Patient Advocacy
**Client-Centered Service
**Practice Philosophy and Values
**Continuous Quality Improvement (CQI)
**The Power of the Entire Healthcare Delivery Team

EFFECTIVE TEACHING

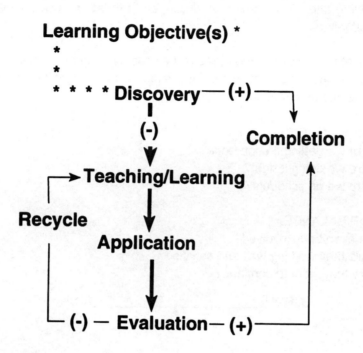

Learning Objective(s) *
   *
   *
  * * * * **Discovery** ── (+) ──┐
         |
       (-)   **Completion**
       ↓
┌──► **Teaching/Learning**
Recycle
| **Application**
|
└── (-) ── **Evaluation** ── (+) ──

(-)   They don't know it yet!

(+)   They show a good understanding of it!

Learning Objectives are for the trainer, not the participants. If participants repli-cate the learning objectives (without being told) after teaching/learning, then effective teaching has occurred.

* * *Minidiscoveries should recur continually during teaching/learning with the facilitated discussion method of sharing knowledge.*

EVALUATING

The goal is to provide positive suggestions for growth and improvement. Critiques, exams, and appraisals must give way to coaching and persuading, to vision building and reinforcement of values, and to performance planning rather than fear of failure.

The values of the individual, the ethics of the situation, and the values of the practice need to be the consistent criteria for evaluation. In this light the six basic leadership questions that need to be answered are:

TASK BALANCE:
   * Are we getting the job done?
   * Are we doing it right?
   * Are we on schedule?

GROUP BALANCE:
   * Is everybody involved?
   * Are they working well and satisfied?
   * Do they want to continue?

GROUP_____TASK
                    ▲

Evaluation, with reflective questions geared to the future, helps the leader keep operational and emotional balance within the group dynamics.

Keep the group together and get the job done—that's all you need to do.

To a caring leader, evaluation is a continuous process. Do it right, for the right reasons, at the right time; keep it positive and make it a building experience.

SITUATIONAL LEADERSHIP

STYLES OF THE LEADER

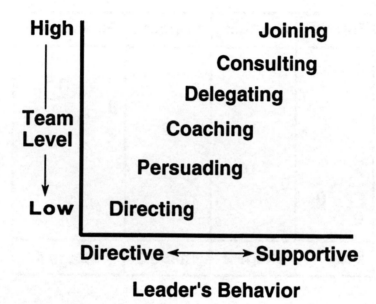

Leader's Behavior

Group Level = development of person
    Low = eager but not able
    Medium = not motivated but knows how
    Medium-high = willing and able to repeat
    High = creative, willing, and able

    Leader's Style = response to group needs*
    Directive = involvement with self and task
    Supportive = involvement with others

*The skilled leader matches the group development needs with the task (see reflecting, fostering group development, and forming personal relationships skills) and adjusts his or her personal approach accordingly.

GROUP DEVELOPMENT

STAGES OF GROUP DEVELOPMENT

Forming	Storming	Norming	Performing
* * * * 0 0	* 0 * 0 * * *	0 0 * * *	* 0 0 * 0 * *
Stage 1	**Stage 2**	**Stage 3**	**Stage 4**

* = relationships (morale)
0 = task/skill effectiveness

Stage 1 = high relationships, low task effectiveness

Stage 2 = lowest relationships while effectiveness begins to increase

Stage 3 = relationships improving, task effectiveness getting better

Stage 4 = high relationships and highest task effectiveness

PERSONAL RELATIONSHIPS

The previous diagram, "Stages of Group Development," should be overlaid with the Practicing Situational Leadership diagram, "Styles of a Leader." The leader's techniques should vary, from directive communication to supportive interaction, with the needs of the group. In the beginning staff members require a very directive training style; then they need to be persuaded they own the job. After they accept ownership, they should be coached to refine their skills and further build their confidence before delegation occurs. Once delegation occurs, don't take it back—just become their consultant.

Previous experiences, bias, and prejudice exist as barriers. A caring leader is a barrier buster! Techniques include one-on-one time investment, attentive listening, expression of personal feelings, behavior awareness (self and others), honesty, accessibility, follow-through, empathy, patience, and quick forgiveness.

In simpler terms, a leader needs:

Caring, Understanding, and Commitment

A veterinary practice needs the uncommon leader, one who seeks barriers to break them down, who opens the program to others, and who strives to help each person exceed his or her own, as well as outside, expectations. Coaching, counseling, and performance planning—not performance appraisals—are essential elements of building a group and maintaining good personal relationships within the practice team.

The leader is accountable for change management, and for the environment that allows everyone to contribute and participate.

Change = Dissatisfaction/Desire × Participative Process × Model < Costs

Albert Schweitzer once said:

I do not know what your destiny will be, but one thing I know: the only ones among you who will be really happy are those who have sought and found how to serve.

INTERNAL PRACTICE PROMOTIONS

THE INTERNAL MARKETING PROCESS

Patient, client, community perceptions + Perceptions of staff, associates, and referring colleagues + Staff attitudes, knowledge, performance commitment, and pride

→ INTERNAL MARKETING STRATEGY →

Complete staff acceptance and knowledge of services, changes, and offerings + perceptions, attitudes, vision, and performance commitment

SALES-MINDEDNESS

→ + →

CLIENT CONSCIOUSNESS

More returning clients and patients + Improved healthcare + Satisfied clients, better bottom line and happier team

Internal marketing boils down to seven truths:

1. The human resources of a practice are the primary market for the practice. If you can't get the staff on your side, the clients will not become satisfied users of the services offered.

2. The staff must understand why they are expected to perform in a certain manner and why you need their support inside and outside the practice.

3. You must convince your staff of the value of the services offered if you want them to support the services. Clients believe employees have the inside scoop.

4. Employees deliver your services. As a team, they need to grasp your expectations, or the intended services will never effectively reach the client.

5. Selling to staff members is a prerequisite for selling to clients. Staff must share in the dream, the vision, and the beliefs of the practice.

6. You must continually motivate and train the paraprofessional staff to extend to clients the communication, compassion, respect, courtesy, and attention your customers deserve and expect.

7. You must strive to attract and retain excellent staff members if you want to attract and retain loyal clients.

CONTINUOUS QUALITY IMPROVEMENT (CQI)

In developing an action plan to confront the habits that a practice needs to change to advance into CQI, there are five truths that must be accepted:

1. There is no more time in any day.
2. Quality occurs after expectations are met.
3. Prevention will lead to quality.
4. Fear of failure prevents quality growth and change.
5. Nonconformity is the price of quality.

There are many ways to describe CQI, but one of the best is to understand the elements that must be put in place by the leadership *before* attempting to start the CQI process; these can be called the pillars of CQI:

THE PILLARS OF CQI—THE FOUNDATION OF THE FUTURE

TRUST IN VALUES	COMMITMENT	ACCOUNTABILITY	RECOGNITION	TRAINING	COMMUNICATION	REMINDERS	EXPECTATIONS	EVALUATION	PROBLEM SOLVING

The *L* in "quality" stands for leadership. One hospital, which accepted the idea that clients perceive pride as quality, and that perception can differentiate a practice, redefined "pride" as its core value by replacing the letters with words:

Patient. The patient always comes first ... and first, do no harm.
Respect. Mutual respect among the team, and consideration for the client and the patient, are primary.
Innovation. Each employee is hired to solve problems, not just to do a job.
Dedication. The quality outcome of every encounter should be everyone's goal.
Excellence. Competency is the best possible performance.

Another practice used the following adage to instill the CQI philosophy within its staff:

Because I dissent, I am not disloyal ...
Because I differ, I am not disloyal ...
Because I care, I will challenge assumptions.

SETTING THE EXAMPLE

A POEM
(author unknown)

I'd rather see a sermon than hear one—any day.

I'd rather one should walk with me rather than merely show the way.

The eye's a better pupil and more willing than the ear;

Fine counsel is confusing, but example is always clear.

The best of all preachers are the men who live their creeds,

For to see the good in action is what everybody needs.

I can say, I'll learn how to do it if you'll let me see it done;

I can watch your hand in action though your tongue too fast may run.

Although lectures you deliver may be very wise and true,

I'd rather learn my lesson by observing what you do;

For I may misunderstand you and the fine advice you give,

But it's not misunderstanding how you act and how you live.

GLOSSARY

(or A Rose by Any Other Name ... Is Confusing.)

The following glossary includes of words from this book and other helpful (and sometimes reworded) terms from *What Every Supervisor Should Know*, by Lester R. Bittel and John K. Newstrom (see the Suggested Reading for this and other readings).

A

active listening: The conscious effort to secure information of all kinds; involves giving the speaker full attention, listening intently and being alert to any clues of spoken or unspoken meaning or resistance, and actively seeking to keep the conversation open and satisfying to the speaker.

adminis-trivia: Catchphrase for administrative trivia.

accountability: An organizational obligation held by a team member, generally with a clearly defined outcome.

appraisal interview: A meeting held between a supervisor and an employee to review the employee's performance rating and, using that evaluation as a basis, to discuss the overall quality of the employee's work and methods for improving it, if necessary; should be replaced by performance planning once CQI is understood.

authority: The legitimate power to ensure that other people work for the good of the practice and can obtain resources from it to achieve desired outcomes.

B

behavior: The actions people take, or the things they say, while coping with other people, problems, opportunities, and situations.

body language: Nonverbal body movements, facial expressions, or gestures that may project and reveal underlying attitudes and sentiments; may convey a message similar to, or different from, the words used.

brainstorming: A group approach to generate ideas that encourages free association of ideas among participants, forbids negative judgments, and generates a maximum number of ideas in a short period of time.

budget: A planning and reporting system for operating programs and results, as well as for costs and expenses, that incorporates many standards into a single dynamic document.

C

catchment area: Primary geographical area served by an institution; demographic area from which clients come.

commitment: In the practice team it is the investment by the individual (not monetary) in the purpose, job role, and feedback process to enhance operational effectiveness.

communication method: The form or technique by which information is communicated, such as attitude, performance, appearance, speech, demonstration, or deed (conversation, discussion, dialogue, book, telephone, recording, radio, public address system, or television).

communication process: The verbal and nonverbal giving and receiving of information and understanding as a result of thinking, doing, observing, talking, listening, writing, and reading; exchange between two or more people, leading to a desired action or attitude.

core values: Those personal standards of excellence and philosophy of operations that underlie all decisions; inviolate beliefs of a leader in which others can also depend.

CQI: Continuous Quality Improvement—a change enhancement and client service movement in healthcare delivery.

D

decision making: The part of the problem-solving process that entails evaluating alternative solutions and making a choice among them.

delegation: The assignment to others of organizational responsibilities or obligations along with appropriate practice authority, power, and rights.

division of work: The principle that performance is more efficient when a large job is broken down into smaller, specialized jobs.

E

employee-centered supervision: Management emphasis on genuine concern and respect for staff members and on maintaining effective relationships within a work group.

employee counseling: A task-oriented, problem-solving technique that features an empathic, interactive discussion that emphasizes listening and is aimed at helping a team member cope with some specific aspect of his or her practice life.

employee turnover: A measure of how many people come to work for an organization and do not remain employed by that organization, for whatever reason.

F

facilitating: Assisting and guiding others in their efforts to perform their jobs rather than emphasizing orders and instructions.

feedback: The return of part of the output to the input of a mechanism, process, or system; informative reaction or response.

free association of ideas: The unconscious ability of the mind to visualize relationships between seemingly different objects and ideas ("brainstorming").

G

grapevine: Informal network that staff members use to convey information of interest to them; fast, but lacks a high degree of accuracy and reliability.

group dynamics: The interaction among members of a work group and concurrent changes in their attitudes, behavior, and relationships; similarly, the interaction (in changing attitudes, behavior, and relationships) between a work group and others outside the group.

H

halo effect: A generalization whereby one aspect of performance, or a single quality of an individual's nature, is allowed to overshadow everything else about that person.

healthcare: The medical, dental, or veterinary delivery of services, products, and empathy.

human relations management: An approach that seeks to stimulate cooperation on the basis of an understanding of, and genuine concern for, staff members as individuals and as critical elements of a work group.

I

infinity model: A leadership and management single-flow diagram; a process, not a program; a total commitment by the leader as a beginning, but has no end.

inner strength: Those internal values and beliefs a person possesses that allows them to be confident and determined in outward activities.

J

jargon: The technical terminology or characteristic idiom of a special activity or group; something used within a practice team but seldom appropriate for use with clients or outside the practice.

job aids: Materials placed on or near the work area to help employees remember key points (what to do and how to do it) and perform effectively.

job role: The team member's part in the practice's operational environment.

L

leader: Someone who gives credit and takes blame, gets things done through other people.

litigious: Inclined toward involvement in lawsuits.

M

management development: A systematic program to improve the knowledge, attitudes, and skills of supervisors and managers.

manager: An individual who plans, organizes, directs, and controls the work of others in an organization.

mentor: A knowledgeable, often influential, individual who takes an interest in, and advises, another person to assist in making that person successful.

modeling: The process in which a skilled co-worker or supervisor demonstrates the performance of a key job skill and simultaneously explains the steps involved and the reasons for doing them; in management, also a graphic representation of a system.

motivation: What impels a person to behave in a certain manner in order to satisfy highly individual needs for survival, security, companionship, respect, achievement, power, growth, and a sense of personal worth.

O

objectives: Also referred to as goals and standards; the short-term and long-term targets toward which an organization strives.

ogre: The doctor after a 22-hour shift.

outer strength: Those elements of management and personality that are displayed to others in the practice's operational environment.

P

participation: The technique by which team members share work-related information, responsibilities, decisions, or all three; may be used to determine the way a job should be performed, how a group should divide the work, and what work goals should be.

patient advocate: One who speaks for what the animal needs rather than using need-to-sell or fear-to-offer habits; one who accepts the Lord's command to Noah as part of the veterinary calling.

performance appraisal: A formal and systematic outdated evaluation scoring system to grade how well a person is performing his or her work to a static standard; in healthcare replaced by CQI and performance planning.

performance planning: A dynamic process whereby 90-day goals and the measurement(s) of success are jointly agreed upon by an individual and his or her mentor, then implemented; efforts evaluated both during in-process learning as well as after the 90 days.

personality: An individual's unique way of behaving and of seeing and interpreting the actions of other people and events; shaped by heredity, parents' beliefs, upbringing, work experiences, and many other factors.

policies: Broad guidelines, philosophy, or principles established by a practice to support its organizational goals.

practice owner: In charge of and responsible for the performance of the team; establishes broad plans, objectives, and general policies.

proactive: Using previous learning, recall, and tenacity to prevent or resolve a challenge *before* others can become reactionary.

problem solving: The process whereby, when a gap occurs between expected and actual conditions or results, the positions are analyzed systematically in order to find and remedy the causes.

procedures: Minimum standards prescribed by management for proper and consistent efforts, sequences, and channels.

productivity: The measure of effectiveness that compares the value of outputs from an operation with the cost of the resources used.

purpose: Most often defined in terms of values, mission, and/or philosophy within a practice; the hub around which all else evolves to make a team effective and help them grasp why they exist as a team.

Q

quality assurance: Establishing milestones and outcome accountabilities for a plan and spot-checking measurements of success toward the end result(s).

quality control: An aggregate of activities designed to ensure that a process is followed with a high degree of consistency and procedural accuracy.

quality of work life: The idea that work must be rewarding materially, psychologically, and spiritually to the person performing it.

quick fix: An expedient, often inadequate, solution to a problem.

R

regulations: Special rules, orders, and controls set by an authority to restrict the conduct of individuals or organizations.

responsibility: A duty or obligation to perform a prescribed task or service or to attain a specified objective.

S

satisfaction: The state that exists when truly motivating factors are provided, such as interesting and challenging work, full use of one's capabilities, and recognition for achievement.

stasis: Act or condition of standing or stopping; in healthcare it equals death.

stress: On- or off-job pressures that place a burden on an individual's physical, mental, or nervous system.

supervisor: Manager or coordinator in charge of the activities of a group; directs work procedures, issues oral and written orders and instructions, assigns duties to workers, examines work for quality and neatness, maintains harmony among workers, and adjusts errors and complaints.

synergy: Combined action or force that is greater than the sum of its elements.

system: An interrelated set of elements that function as a whole.

T

TQM: Total Quality Management—improvement movement in industry.

TQS/TMS: Total Quality Service/Total Management Service—copycat management ideas of lateral organizations trying to reinvent TQM/CQI.

U

unity of direction: The principle that there should be a set of goals and objectives that unifies the activities of everyone in an organization.

V

values: A set of personal beliefs that forms the foundation for life decisions.

W

work: That four-letter word for employment that provides the means to pay the bills.

SUGGESTED READING

Author's Note: The bold references form the minimum library to collect as you seek the leadership advantage.

Leadership Skills

Atchison, T.A. *Turning Healthcare Leadership Around.* San Francisco: Jossey-Bass, 1991.

Boone, Mary E. *Leadership and the Computer.* Rocklin, Calif.: Prima, 1991.

Carnegie, Dale. *The Leader in You.* New York: Simon and Schuster, 1993.

Covey, Stephen R. *Seven Habits of Highly Effective People.* New York: Simon and Schuster, Fireside, 1990.

Drucker, Peter F. *Managing for Results: Economic Tasks and Risk-taking.* New York: Harper and Row, 1964.

Juran, J.M. *Juran on Leadership for Quality.* New York: Free Press, 1989.

Pagonis, William G. *Moving Mountains.* Waco, Tex.: Baylor University Extract, 1985.

Best Business Reading

Bennis, Warren, and Bert Nanus. *Leaders, Strategies for Taking Charge.* New York: Harper and Row, 1985.

Block, Peter. *The Empowered Manager: Positive Political Skills at Work.* San Francisco: Jossey-Bass, 1987.

Peters, Tom. *Liberation Management: Necessary Disorganization for the Nanosecond Nineties.* New York: A. A. Knopf, 1992.

Senge, Peter M. *The Fifth Discipline: The Art and Practice of the Learning Organization.* New York: Doubleday, 1990.

***Successful Financial Management.* Denver, Colo.: American Animal Hospital Association, 1987.**

Sharpen Your Personal Skills

Bracey, Hyler, Jack Rosenblum, Aubrey Sanford, and Roy Trueblood. *Managing from the Heart.* New York: Delacorte Press, 1990.

Gottlieb, Marvin, and William J. Healy. *Making Deals: The Business of Negotiating.* New York: New York Institute of Finance, 1990.

Heirs, Ben, with Peter Farrell. *The Professional Decision Thinker: America's New Management and Education Priority.* New York: Dodd Mead, 1987.

Nelson, Robert B. *Empowering Employees Through Delegation.* Burr Ridge, Ill.: Irwin Professional Publications, 1994.

Seiwert, Lothar J. *Time Is Money: Save It.* Homewood, Ill.: Dow Jones-Irwin, 1989.

Webber, Ross Arkell. *Becoming a Courageous Manager: Overcoming Career Problems of New Managers.* Englewood Cliffs, N.J.: Prentice Hall, 1991.

Get Ready for Tomorrow

Drucker, Peter F. *Managing for the Future: The 1990s and Beyond.* New York: Dutton, 1992.

_____. *Post Capitalistic Society.* New York: Harper Collins, 1993.

Dychtwald, Ken, and Joe Flower. *Age Wave: The Challenges and Opportunities of an Aging America.* Los Angeles: J.P. Tarcher, 1989.

Jamieson, David, and Julie O'Mara. *Managing Workforce 2000: Gaining the Di-*

versity Advantage. San Francisco: Jossey-Bass, 1991.

McNally, David. *Even Eagles Need a Push.* New York: Bantam Doubleday Dell, 1990.

Schwartz, Peter. *The Art of the Long View.* New York: Doubleday, 1991.

Management Skills That Work

Jellison, Jerald M. *Overcoming Resistance: A Practical Guide to Producing Change in the Work Place.* New York: Simon and Schuster, 1993.

Kaplan, Robert E. *Beyond Ambition: How Driven Managers Can Lead Better and Live Better.* San Francisco: Jossey-Bass, 1991.

Katzenbach, Jon R., and Douglas K. Smith. *The Wisdom of Teams: Creating the High-Performance Organization.* Boston: Harvard Business School Press, 1993.

LeBoeuf, Michael. *The Greatest Management Principle in the World, GMP.* New York: Berkley Books, 1985.

New Tactics for Managers

Bardwick, Judith M. *Danger in the Comfort Zone: From Boardroom to Mailroom—How to Break the Entitlement Habit That's Killing American Business.* New York: AMACOM, 1991.

Bittel, Lester R., and John W. Newstrom. *What Every Supervisor Should Know,* 6th ed. New York: McGraw-Hill, 1990.

Horton, R., and Peter C. Reid. *Beyond the Trust Gap: Forging a New Partnership Between Managers and Their Employees.* Homewood, Ill.: Business One Irwin, 1991.

Leebov, Wendy, and Gail Scott. *Healthcare Managers in Transition.* San Francisco: Jossey-Bass, 1990.

Shonk, James H. *Team-Based Organizations: Developing a Successful Team Environment.* Homewood, Ill.: Business One Irwin, 1992.

Reach Your Customers

Albrecht, Karl, and Lawrence J. Bradford. *The Service Advantage: How to Identify and Fulfill Customer Needs.* Homewood, Ill.: Dow Jones-Irwin, 1990.

Carlzon, Jan. *Moments of Truth.* Cambridge, Mass.: Ballinger, 1987.

Connellan, Thomas K., and Ron Zemke. *Sustaining Knock Your Socks Off Service.* New York: AMACOM, 1993.

Davidow, William H., and Bro Uttal. *Total Customer Service: The Ultimate Weapon.* New York: Harper and Row, 1989.

LeBoeuf, Michael. *How to Win Customers and Keep Them for Life.* New York: Berkley Books, 1987.

Learning to Motivate People

Albrecht, Karl, with Steven Albrecht. *The Creative Corporation.* Homewood, Ill.: Dow Jones-Irwin, 1987.

Kravetz, Dennis J. *The Human Resources Revolution: Implementing Progressive Management Practices for Bottom-Line Success.* San Francisco: Jossey-Bass, 1988.

Levering, Robert. *A Great Place to Work.* New York: Random House, 1988.

Matejka, Ken E. *Why This Horse Won't Drink: How to Win and Keep Employee Commitment.* New York: American Management Association, 1991.

Roethlisberger, Fritz Jules. *Management and Morale.* Cambridge, Mass.: Harvard University Press, 1941.

von Oech, Roger. *A Kick in the Seat of the Pants.* Harper and Row, Perennial Library, 1986.

Winning Sales Techniques

Finch, Lloyd. *Telephone Courtesy and Customer Service*. Los Altos, Calif.: Crisp Publications, 1987.

Gerson, Richard. *Beyond Customer Service: Keeping Customers for Life*. Los Altos, Calif.: Crisp, 1992.

Hanan, Mack. *Successful Market Penetration: How to Shorten the Sales Cycle by Making the First Sale the First Time*. New York: American Management Association, 1987.

Laughlin, Chuck, and Karen Sage, with Marc Bockman. *Samurai Selling: The Ancient Art of Service in Sales*. New York: St. Martin's, 1993.

Scott, Dru. *Customer Satisfaction*. Los Altos, Calif.: Crisp, 1988.

Willingham, Ron. *Integrity Selling: How to Succeed in Selling in the Competitive Years Ahead*. Garden City, N.Y.: Doubleday, 1987.

Wilson, Larry, with Hersch Wilson. *Changing the Game: The New Way to Sell*. New York: Simon and Schuster, Fireside, 1988.

Communication

Bazerman, Max H., and Margaret A. Neale. *Negotiating Reality*. New York: Free Press, 1992.

Decker, Bert, with Jim Denney. *You've Got to Be Believed to Be Heard*. New York: St. Martin's, 1992.

Frank, Milo O. *How to Get Your Point Across in Thirty Seconds or Less*. New York: Simon and Schuster, 1986.

McCallister, Linda. *I Wish I'd Said That: How to Talk Your Way Out of Trouble and into Success*. New York: Wiley, 1992.

Mosvick, K., and Robert B. Nelson. *We've Got to Start Meeting Like This: A Guide to Successful Business Meeting Management*. Glenview, Ill.: Scott, Foresman, 1987.

Rafe, Stephen C. *How to Be Prepared to Think on Your Feet*. New York: Harper Business, 1990.

Lightning Source UK Ltd.
Milton Keynes UK
UKOW02f1533180214

226648UK00007B/107/P